Patient and Public Involvement Toolkit

Patient and Public Involvement Toolkit

BY

Julia Cartwright

Director, Flex Business Consulting Ltd
Chair, The Community Partnership Forum,
The Better Healthcare Programme for Banbury & Surrounding Areas

Sally Crowe

Director, Crowe Associates Ltd
Chair, The James Lind Alliance

EDITORS

Carl Heneghan
Rafael Perera
Douglas Badenoch

BMJ|Books

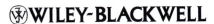

A John Wiley & Sons, Ltd., Publication

BMJ Books is an imprint of BMJ Publishing Group Limited, used under licence by Blackwell Publishing which was acquired by John Wiley & Sons in February 2007. Blackwell's publishing programme has been merged with Wiley's global Scientific, Technical and Medical business to form Wiley-Blackwell.

Registered office: John Wiley & Sons Ltd, The Atrium, Southern Gate, Chichester, West Sussex, PO19 8SQ, UK

Editorial offices: 9600 Garsington Road, Oxford, OX4 2DQ, UK
                     The Atrium, Southern Gate, Chichester, West Sussex, PO19 8SQ, UK
                     111 River Street, Hoboken, NJ 07030-5774, USA

For details of our global editorial offices, for customer services and for information about how to apply for permission to reuse the copyright material in this book please see our website at www.wiley.com/wiley-blackwell

Library of Congress Cataloging-in-Publication Data
Cartwright, Julia.
    Patient and public involvement toolkit / by Julia Cartwright, Sally Crowe; editors, Carl Heneghan, Rafael Perera, Douglas Badenoch.
        p. ; cm.
    Includes bibliographical references.
    ISBN 978-1-4051-9910-0
    1. Patient participation.   2. Health planning.   I. Crowe, Sally.   II. Heneghan, Carl.   III. Perera, Rafael.   IV. Badenoch, Douglas.   V. Title.
    [DNLM: 1. Patient Participation–methods–Great Britain–Handbooks.   2. Consumer Participation–Great Britain–Handbooks.   3. Delivery of Health Care–methods–Great Britain–Handbooks.   W 49]
    R727.42.C37 2011
    362.1–dc22
                                        2010038256
ISBN: 978-1-4051-9910-0

A catalogue record for this book is available from the British Library.

Set in 9/7 pt Frutiger Light by Toppan Best-set Premedia Limited

This book is published in the following electronic formats: ePDF 9781444328387; Wiley Online Library 9781444328370

1   2011

Contents

Foreword

"Involve, Engage, Empower" – how often have we heard those words used in health care planning, only to find that they really mean nothing? This book is the opposite of that. It dares the reader to mean business with patient involvement, engagement, and – most dangerous of all – empowerment. It leaves you with no excuse for not getting on with it, because everything you need is here, bar a tin of shoe polish.

The reason that Julia Cartwright writes with such clarity and authority is that she has actually made this happen. Uniquely, she brought together all the stakeholders in the locality where I practised as a GP for 31 years, and by a mixture of personal skill, energy and endless patience achieved agreement on issues which had plagued us for most of that period. Julia's co-author, Sally Crowe, is helping to set the agenda for a genuinely patient-centred model of health care through her work with the James Lind Alliance, and its programme of identifying the research that is needed to support this.

When they tell you how to give a presentation, how to deal with unhelpful contributors, how to listen and how to react, do as they say: they know their business.

This is difficult work, and this book could not be more timely. General practitioners driven to despair by having to commission local care within a dwindling budget will find it full of advice on how to share such decisions meaningfully with local patients and politicians. The empowerment of patients is an inevitable part not just of current political rhetoric, but future reality.

User-driven health care is on the way: it challenges each one of us, either as a user or a professional, or both. This jargon-free book, with its excellent links, its clear analysis and its brilliantly practical approach is the best tool I know of to address this coming reality.

Richard Lehman
Medical Adviser,
Health Experiences Research Group,
Oxford University
20 Nov 2010

CHAPTER 1
Introduction

The toolkit series

The 'toolkit' series encompasses a number of books and a website published by Blackwell. The concept behind the books is to make complex health care topics accessible and easy to understand to those who need them, particularly:

- health care students
- clinicians
- users of health care research
- researchers
- commissioners of health services and research.

This book is the fourth in the current series of toolkits, which also includes the *Evidence-Based Medicine Toolkit*, the *Statistics Toolkit* and the *Searching Toolkit*. The writing team for this book is Julia Cartwright and Sally Crowe, both experts in patient and public involvement (PPI). The editing team is Douglas Badenoch, Carl Heneghan and Rafael Perrera.

Aim of this toolkit

> The purpose of this toolkit is to help you undertake effective patient and public involvement (PPI) in your work. This could be clinical research, service redesign, policy development or commissioning activities.

This book will take you through the journey of involving patients, carers and the public, with chapters that address specific and important stages of the journey. At the end of each chapter there will be a key points summary table. A list of icons used throughout the book is given on page 14.

We have created resource lists at the end of each section that will help you locate useful resources. While all of the resources were checked before publication, PPI is an evolving and fast-moving world, with new groups, resources and ideas becoming available all of the time. Since going into production, the UK government has issued its White Paper on health

Patient and Public Involvement Toolkit, 1st edition. By © J. Cartwright, S. Crowe, R. Perera, C. Heneghan & D. Badenoch. Published 2011 by Blackwell Publishing Ltd.

(Department of Health, 2010), *Equity and Excellence*. 'No decision about me without me' is the strap line for this policy document which aims to put patients at the heart of decision making in the NHS. This toolkit is therefore a timely resource for those individuals who need to make PPI happen. http://www.dh.gov.uk/en/Publicationsandstatistics/Publications/ PublicationsPolicyAndGuidance/DH_117353.

Why have a PPI toolkit?

PPI is becoming much more integrated into service development at every level of health care, and increasingly is a common part of clinical health research. Despite these advances, PPI is often haphazard and inconsistent, with a plethora of individual but unconnected activities.

Therefore, we decided there is a need for a clear, simple toolkit that will help you to:

- **Identify** the purpose and useful outcomes of PPI.
- **Understand** how to run effective PPI programmes and how to engage constructively with patients.
- **Clarify** to those involved in a PPI programme what to expect from their involvement and how to make their voices heard.

EFFECTIVE PPI CHECKLIST
Some of the most effective PPI happens when:

1 There is a clear understanding of what is needed to enable effective involvement.
2 There is recognition of the likely barriers to effective engagement.
3 The purpose and benefits of involvement are clear to everyone.
4 There is attention to detail.

The language of PPI

One of the problems in PPI is the complexity of the language that is used. This has been recognized at the highest level:

The conflation of these distinct terms and the confusion about the purpose of involvement has led to muddled initiatives and uncertainty about what should be done to achieve effective PPI.
UK Parliament, House of Commons Health Committee Report 2007

Getting started
What is PPI?

Healthcare professionals working together with patients and the public to improve the health communities they serve.

> **health professional** A health professional is an organization, team or person who delivers health care in a professional manner to any individual in need of health care services.

Why do PPI?
- To improve **access** to health services.
- To have a better **informed** public.
- To improve the **quality** of health care.
- To make better use of health care **resources**.
- To improve how health services are **measured** and **evaluated**.

Who can benefit from PPI?
- **Patients** if they see their views being considered and used to improve the quality of care for other patients.
- **Health researchers** if they see that the quality of their research design and outputs are improved by working with patients from the outset.
- **Health service managers** if the standards of service they design are patient friendly and reduce the level of inappropriate admissions to hospital.
- **Health professionals** if they see a reduction in attendance at specialist clinics because patients can better self-care at home.
- **Public** if they see that decisions about health care and services are transparent and accountable.

For this toolkit we use the following terms throughout:

Term	Definition
INVOLVE	To Inform. To consult. *'Surely we are at the heart of care and treatment? My experiences can help services improve'*
ENGAGE	To partner. To work directly with. *'I want staff to think about opportunities for PPI at the start of all projects'*
EMPOWER	To place authority for final decision making in the hands of the patient or the public. *'We would like to see more patients and public at senior management meetings and having a real input to future strategy'*

Sections will be colour coded throughout to help you see what level of PPI is being described or suggested.

The following words are prohibited from this toolkit:

- **Participatory** – we will write about working with people.
- **Stakeholder** – we will write about patients or public.
- **Client** – we will talk about patients or public.
- **Dialogue** – we will write about talking to patients or public.
- **Facilitate** – we will write about working together and sharing.
- **Partnership** – we will write about doing things together.
- **Lay** – we will write about patients and the public.

For further words that should not be used when communicating with patients and the public go to:
www.idea.gov.uk/idk/core/page.do?pageId=17636724

KEY TERMS

patient People who are under the care of clinical services, or have recently used these services.

carers People who care for others in an 'unpaid' and non-professional capacity.

public People who are not under the care of clinical services but who may have a view on those services.

patient involvement Involving people who have used health services.

public involvement Involving people as citizens who may or may not have used services.

National Health Service (NHS) The NHS is the name used to refer to the publically funded healthcare systems in Great Britain.

Primary Care Trusts (PCT) PCTs are part of the NHS. They provide some primary and community services and commission secondary care services.

Levels of PPI

Involvement is often referred to at different levels, suggesting different types of activity and outcome. In this book we will use involvement (rose), engagement (pink) and empowerment (red).

The following examples will help you to understand the different levels of involvement using different case studies.

- Designing hospital signs.
- Redesigning an outpatient service.
- A collaborative research proposal in cancer.
- Developing a patient information resource.
- A local public awareness campaign for flu.
- Commissioning a primary care service for mild to moderate depression.
- Determining local health priorities.

They illustrate the different settings for PPI involvement and show you how the different levels of PPI can work in practice. Without recognizing the different impacts PPI can have on health care, it may be difficult for you to envisage how you might incorporate it into the development of new services, research proposals and in determining priorities for local health services.

Each example is described from both patient and public perspectives. These themes will be repeated throughout the toolkit; it might be worth referring to them when you are about to investigate your own patient and public involvement project.

Designing hospital signs

INVOLVEMENT

Members of
the public

An information leaflet is displayed in public areas informing the community that the local hospital will have a new sign and signage

Patients

The local hospital patient user's group is asked where they think the new hospital signs need to be located

ENGAGEMENT

Members of
the public

The communications director arranges a presentation of new designs for hospital signs to public bodies such as county and district councils.

Feedback from the event is used to inform the final version of the hospital signage

Patients

The communications director arranges a presentation to patient groups showing them proposed designs for the new hospital signage

Feedback from the presentation is used to inform the final versions of the location and design

EMPOWERMENT

Members of
the public

The Health Overview & Scrutiny Committee has received complaints that the local hospital signage is difficult to read and understand. This makes access to the hospital difficult for patients

They raise the issue at a hospital trust board meeting which has public access and agree that they will work with local community groups to prepare designs which are user friendly, welcoming and correctly located

They will conduct a 'before and after' survey to test their methodology to ensure that they add to the evidence base of positive user involvement improving access to health services

Patients

The local hospital user group representative informs the hospital governing board that 45% of patients surveyed said that they could not read the hospital signage

The user group, who has a trained expert in health communication design as a member, would therefore work with a team of patients, public bodies and a design team to work up a proposal for new, user-friendly signage

Redesigning an outpatient service

Public

Posters and leaflets displayed in public areas (and on the relevant web pages) inform the outpatient service users that changes are coming

The Local Involvement Network is contacted about plans and invited to participate

Previous satisfaction surveys and monitoring information are reviewed for feedback on out patient service

Patients

The local hospital patient user group is asked what sort of out patient service they would like

This could be achieved within an existing meeting, a specific focus group or with a short survey (web and/or paper based)

Public

A specific event is held showcasing ideas for service development, with an open invitation and targeting those who have already contributed

Feedback from the event is used to inform the specification of service

Patients

Feedback is arranged to the patient user group from the event and final specifications are discussed

Specific patient groups with specific needs are targeted for feedback

Public

Members of the public who have previously been involved in the consultation are invited to view and test the new service – and give feedback in its early stages

Patients

Two members of the patient group attend project guidance meetings to ensure that patient and public feedback is integral to the design and implementation of the service

These members are also involved in site visits and other practical arrangements for the changes

INVOLVEMENT

ENGAGEMENT

EMPOWERMENT

A collaborative research proposal in cancer

INVOLVEMENT

Members of
the public

The public may be appropriately involved if the research concerns the prevention of cancer and addressing lifestyle factors. Raising awareness of the need for the research project by distributing posters to hospitals

Patients

Finding local support groups that might be interested in an exploratory meeting/workshop to outline the nature of the research and how current and past cancer patients can help

ENGAGEMENT

Members of
the public

As below

Patients

Working with patients' groups to:
- Monitor and steer the project
- Define the research question
- Ask what outcomes should be measured in the study
- Assess the viability of the research protocol
- Assist with networking and information to engage/recruit patients to the study
- Share the results with the study population

EMPOWERMENT

Members of
the public

As below

Patients

Members of patient groups may be recruited as co-researchers with roles such as:
- Monitoring and steering the project
- Helping with gathering data
- Gathering data with support from other researchers
- Analysing data with researchers
- Providing commentary on outcomes and results
- Helping with dissemination and translational aspects of research results.

Developing a patient information resource

INVOLVEMENT

Members of the public

A primary care provider wants to prepare a poster about the benefits of immunization to child health. They design three different posters and take them to a local mother and toddler club and ask the mothers which ones they are most likely to read. From the feedback they receive from the mothers they decide which poster is circulated

Patients

An acute hospital wants to prepare a patient information leaflet on surgical procedures in weight loss surgery. They ask a senior clinician to write the leaflet and then show a draft to their hospital patient panel for comment

ENGAGEMENT

Members of the public

A primary care provider wants to prepare a poster about the benefits of immunization to child health. They know that within certain communities immunization rates are low. They approach a mother and toddler group within such a community and ask the mothers to help design the poster

Patients

Senior clinicians (nurses and doctors) are aware that communicating the different surgical procedures available to weight loss surgery patients can be difficult. The clinicians consider developing visual aids to help the communication process and informed consent

They contact patients who have undergone weight loss surgery and ask them to work with them, a medical designer and a patient advocate if needed, to produce visual aids

EMPOWERMENT

Members of the public

Mothers and health workers within a community with low immunization rates for childhood diseases are concerned at the impact on child health within the community

The mothers and health workers approach their primary care provider and ask to work with them to design a social marketing campaign to increase immunization rates

Patients

A weight loss surgery support group runs a blog for individuals who have either undergone weight loss surgery or who are considering it

Individuals using the blog have commented on the lack of appropriate patient information available on different surgical weight loss methods.

The support group decides to produce its own patient information DVD. They approach the weight loss surgeon at the acute trust, who agrees to work with them to produce the DVD

The DVD is then used by the acute trust

A local public awareness campaign for flu

INVOLVEMENT

Members of the public

Finding out from the public what they need to know about flu, e.g. signs and symptoms, what to do, what not to do, how to communicate risk

Testing these ideas with members of the public to gauge their reaction to and comprehension of the message

Patients

This could be achieved in a focus group. Work with patient groups to alert those at extra risk from flu to ensure that those who need it are immunized quickly. An information meeting, with a panel comprising public members, public health communications experts, primary care, etc., to answer questions

ENGAGEMENT

Members of the public

After agreeing what we need to say and how we will say it, we return to our focus group to get feedback

Identify cultural and communication barriers that might inhibit some people to seek immunization and/or treatment

Patients

Community leaders and influencers may assist communication, especially in communities that are at risk, or for whom English may not be first language, and can help with both the suitability of written material and as local advocates. Develop relationships with patient organizations (of those patients identified as at risk) to use communication materials to best advantage

EMPOWERMENT

Members of the public

Return to community leaders or influencers after the crisis to assess how it was managed and what could be learnt from the experience

This could take place in a meeting or focus group

Patients

Monitoring input on at-risk patients being followed up for immunization and treatment

After the 'crisis' period is over patients can be part of a review process – for lessons learned and how to improve response for next time

Commissioning a primary care service for mild to moderate depression

INVOLVEMENT

Members of the public

Information and invitations are sent by post to target groups who are known to suffer from mild to moderate depression via GP surgeries and primary health care centres

Patients

Make contact with local mental health support groups to establish their interest in getting involved in the project

Gathering existing evidence of service users' experiences of treatment and care for mild to moderate depression

Gathering new data to reflect the gaps in existing evidence; via focus groups, surveys, discussion forum or visiting existing support group meetings and having a conversation

Approach GP Patient Participation Groups to assess their experience of mild to moderate depression

ENGAGEMENT

Members of the public

Working with the public to understand and build into services the problems associated with mild to moderate depression that stop people seeking services, e.g. stigma and shame, etc.

Working with other public service representatives on the role of other forms of treatment such as exercise, relaxation, etc., and how this can be reflected in commissioning

Using local media to gather stories of treatment and care of mild to moderate depression

Patients

Working with patient groups to develop and implement the gathering of new data on primary care services for mild to moderate depression and mapping it across the local area

Analysis of data, feedback on data and implications for services, a workshop with service users, carers, primary care commissioners and mental health professionals participating. Work towards recommendations for commissioning services

EMPOWERMENT

Members of
the public

As below

Patients

Involvement in work to ensure that commissioning plans meet and reflect expected standards and guidance on mild to moderate depression

Involved patients to be part of feedback loop on development of commissioning contract

Review commissioning plans (as part of a working group or other) to ensure that the essence of patient feedback is still maintained in contracts

Contributing to communication (leaflets, web page) that describes the changes to the services commissioned and what patients can expect to receive in treatment and care for mild to moderate depression

Monitoring role – have the commissioned services helped those with mild to moderate depression?

Determining local health priorities

INVOLVEMENT

Members of
the public

Seek the views about health priorities from a range of actual and potential service users

Develop a panel of local people that can be communicated with face to face, by telephone, internet and post

Consider a wider consultation strategy that reaches a significant proportion of the local population

Patients

Identify local patient and support groups

Approach them with the idea for developing health priorities and establish the best ways of communicating with them.

ENGAGEMENT

Members of
the public

Hold open workshops, exhibitions and other events that help people explore, discuss and compare what matters to them in local service improvement

Use voting methods or consensus development methods to help prioritize competing alternatives

Patients

As above, but from a patient perspective

EMPOWERMENT

Members of
the public

Public getting involved in actual commissioning decisions. Acting as advocates for priorities developed by the public. Usually entails reviewing existing priorities and government priorities, assessing available resources in light of local priorities. For those that participate in this more strategic work, there should be appropriate induction and support

Patients

As above, but from a patient perspective

Further reading

Department of Health. *Equity and excellence: liberating the NHS*. London: Department of Health, 2010. www.dh.gov.uk/en/Publicationsandstatistics/Publications/ PublicationsPolicyAndGuidance/DH_117353.

 key message

 tool

 checklist

 PPI examples and case studies

 PPI techniques

 PPI development methods

 summary

CHAPTER 2

What is patient and public involvement?

> **PPI is...**
>
> ...involving people or organizations that have experience of planning, managing and reviewing services
>
> ...involving people or organizations as citizens to ensure public accountability
>
> ...involving people or organizations in choosing priorities for investment and disinvestment
>
> ...involving people or organizations in monitoring the quality of services
>
> ...working with people or organizations that have a particular perspective in the development and implementation (and dissemination) of research
>
> ...commissioning research that reflects the needs and views of the public as well as clinical and scientific perspectives
>
> **PPI isn't...**
>
> ...about patients complying with treatment
>
> ...getting involved in specific decisions about their health care
>
> ...getting people to 'rubber stamp' a decision that has already been made
>
> ...being a subject of a research study
>
> ...being part of a group process but having no real say or power

Why bother with PPI?

PPI in health care usually has one or more of the following objectives:

- Improving information about services.
- Improving access to services.
- Improving the quality of services.

Patient and Public Involvement Toolkit, 1st edition. By © J. Cartwright, S. Crowe, R. Perera, C. Heneghan & D. Badenoch. Published 2011 by Blackwell Publishing Ltd.

- Improving monitoring of services.
- Providing perspectives on the changing needs of patients and the public.
- Increasing recruitment to clinical trials and other studies.
- Improving information about trials and other research.
- Providing a 'critical friend' perspective to projects and programmes, such as capital projects or service redesign.
- Increasing transparency in strategic matters.
- Increasing accountability to local communities.

In addition, for PPI to be effective it has to address the issue of accountability, which can be defined as:

- **Taking into account**: the shaping of activities and priorities (for example through consultation).
- **Giving an account**: explaining actions that have been taken (for example through performance plans).
- **Holding to account**: actions taken by the public and patients once they have heard the account given (for example Overview and Scrutiny Committees).
- **Redress**: a right to redress when services have not been delivered to an appropriate standard.

Why is PPI growing in health and social care?

The journey of health reform is a continuous process and there is no doubt that PPI's place in this reform has evolved in part because of past problems with health care services. These have included organizational failures where unusually high mortality rates or significant patterns of complaints from health service users have been missed.

This has sometimes had tragic consequences, with patients and carers motivated to speak out or get involved so that 'someone else doesn't have to go through what we did'.

Increased public involvement, and a more transparent and open culture of reporting, is likely to result in higher levels of scrutiny of services and challenges to the status quo of health care provision. This can been seen in a positive and constructive light – or perceived as threatening and a 'dumbing down' of the science of health care. Often, PPI is political and challenging.

Consequently, large health organizations are not known for being outward facing. They often have their own cultural identities and 'short-hand' language and while they serve the 'outside' world they rarely interact with it. PPI can help bridge this gap, making links to communities of interest and to the communities that the organization is there to serve.

Early PPI in projects can help identify potential ethical concerns associated with research or in reducing services. It can also find solutions to these problems and help improve the ethical acceptability of decisions. An increased mutual understanding of the pressures of providing 24-hour services or planning care in a time of restricted resources can open up the possibilities for PPI to improve and enhance health and social care.

For example:

- Focus groups of patients can help weigh up the risk–benefit relationships of treatments that are controversial and experimental.
- Public involvement in an audit committee can see hospital data from a different perspective and contribute to critical but creative discussions to improve patient outcomes or efficiency.
- Patient involvement in developing a clinical trial can highlight areas where patients will want explicit information about the benefits and harms of being a research subject.

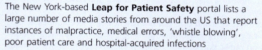

EXAMPLE: PPI IN ACTION
The New York-based **Leap for Patient Safety** portal lists a large number of media stories from around the US that report instances of malpractice, medical errors, 'whistle blowing', poor patient care and hospital-acquired infections

Each item carries a brief explanation, a date of posting, links to the media source and is illustrated with a photograph.

Titles of items currently include: 'When it comes to patient safety, Nevadans are still waiting to join the party'; 'Whistleblower tells of America's hidden nightmare for its sick poor'; and 'Doctor fired over "America Dies on Dunkin" sign'.

[www.leapforpatientsafety.org]

Changes in PPI legislation

The growth in PPI legislation is linked to the growth in citizenship, democracy and rights. This is reflected in the changes to the centres of power within the health and social care system.

Whether through Community Health Councils, Local Involvement Networks or patient forums, patients, carers and the public have gradually been integrated into the planning, commissioning, delivery and evaluation of health care services for some time. For example, in the UK in the past two years there have been moves to make PPI the centre of public service concepts such as Patient Choice and Direct Payments for Services.

The 'customer is king' mantra of business is now filtering into health and social care. Services that are geared more towards those that use them than provide them are the likely future direction.

How does PPI help organizations and services and care change?

For PPI to be effective and helpful, three different elements need to be considered: the consumerist, the democratic and the public health elements.

- **Consumerist element** – this is about ensuring that we provide, as far as possible, the range of services people need in a way people want that is informed by relevant research.
- **Democratic element** – this is about ensuring services are provided fairly, equitably and accountably, in the context of constrained resources.
- **Public health element** – this is recognizing that people have expertise in relation to improving their health as individuals, and collectively as a community.

Public involvement in health care is a prominent policy in countries across the economically developed world. A growing body of academic literature has focused on public participation, often presenting dichotomies between good and bad practice.

Improving health services

In the UK, the NHS Constitution states that the public have the 'right to be involved, directly or through representatives, in the planning of healthcare services, the development and consideration of proposals for changes in the way those services are provided, and in decisions to be made affecting the operation of those services'.

Legislation (Section 242 of the consolidated NHS Act 2007) places a duty on NHS trusts, primary care trusts (PCTs) and strategic health authorities to ensure that patients and the public are involved in service planning and operation, and in the development of proposals for changes in their area.

It also seems sensible that service deliverers are interested in what service users think. PPI activities should generate data about what matters to patients. This data can be '**patient-derived**' (i.e. comes *from* patients directly or indirectly) or '**patient experience data**' (i.e. is *about* people's experiences of services). Data can be used for strategic planning, monitoring and improvement.

You may not need to generate all of your own data – there are plenty of patient and public organizations that act as a window on patient experiences. These can be structured but informal, such as **OUTLET**, or structured and formal such as **HealthTalkOnline**.

Glasgow-based **Outlet** is an internet forum that allows people with mental illness to make contact, compare experiences and offer support.

Four categories of people are invited to register as members:
- parents with mental illness
- children and teenagers of parents with mental illness
- carers of a family member with mental illness
- adults who grew up with a parent with mental illness.

As well as its online forums, Outlet holds virtual gallery space for creative input by children and provides information for patients.

Set up in 2004 by a PhD student at the University of Strathclyde, Outlet also publicizes research projects at the university's departments of psychology and education to which people with mental health problems might wish to offer contributory input.

Outlet does not run any face-to-face meetings.

[www.outlet-scotland.org/website/index.php?option=com_frontpage&Itemid=1]

Healthtalkonline lets you share in other people's experiences of health and illness. You can watch or listen to videos of the interviews, read about people's experiences and find reliable information about conditions, treatment choices and support.

The information on Healthtalkonline is based on qualitative research into patient experiences, led by experts at the University of Oxford. These personal stories of health and illness will enable patients, families and health care professionals to benefit from the experiences of others.

www.healthtalkonline.org

Improving health research

There are other ways that patients, carers and the public can contribute their experiences. They can provide research questions concerning treatment and care that may be missed by more conventional research commissioning and funding programmes. They can peer review research proposals and publications to establish how well the studies take into account the impact on patients.

The involvement of patients in health research is crucial because (Chalmers, 1995):

- it fosters research that is relevant and useful to patients and carers
- the process of involvement encourages a more open-minded approach to what research questions need asking, which forms of health care are worth investigating and which treatment outcomes matter.

The **James Lind Alliance** is a UK-based collaboration of patient, and clinician and research groups that gather data about 'treatment uncertainties'. These are research questions that are not currently answered by up-to-date research. These are published in NHS Evidence – UK DUETs (www.library.nhs.uk/duets/) for research commissioners and funders to take account of.

The James Lind Alliance supports Priority Setting Partnerships to agree the 10 most important of these research questions. These are then promoted by the partnership as priority areas for research. This approach yields priorities that reflect both patients and clinician perspectives and therefore have the potential to have great impact in day-to-day health care (www.lindalliance.org).

As the James Lind Alliance gathers examples of patients and clinicians working together to identify research priorities, an online guidebook describes the principles and process, and has downloadable resources and templates. Visit www.JLAguidebook.org for further information.

Patient and public involvement in clinical research and translational research (helping research have impact at a practical and clinical level) has seen a significant growth in the last 30 years.

Prevailing notions of democracy require that the general public, who ultimately provide funds, should influence research.
Entwistle *et al.* (1998)

PPI in health care research should be considered at all levels of the process. This could include deciding on areas to be researched, helping with the planning and design of research, actually carrying out some of the research (running focus groups for example), reviewing results of research and sharing these widely.

Peer review is an established method for sifting and deciding on good quality and relevant research proposals and policy guidance. PPI in peer review has been successful in UK NHS programmes and in selected UK medical research charities. The key aspect of this type of activity is that peer reviewers are not seen as scientific or medical experts (although they may have related experience) but as providing input about the relevance and pragmatic aspects of the proposals or policy under review.

EXAMPLE: PPI IN RESEARCH

A group of parents with children with a rare and debilitating genetic condition are asked to comment on a trial protocol for a new treatment. The parents meet with the research group and an external facilitator. They first learn about what makes a good research study together, they then hear about the proposed study and work together on the draft protocol (the 'this is how we will do the study' document). They are able to advise the trial team about the likelihood of the protocol being suitable for these children and families to participate in the trial. There is a small population of children with the condition, therefore it is important that as many families as possible are recruited to the trial. The redesigned protocol acknowledges the limitations of families to attend clinics and participate in certain procedures, and promotes more flexibility in the monitoring phase. It is hoped that these changes will enhance recruitment to the trial and reduce potential drop out of children and families.

Notes: *While children are the focus of the trial, it is parents/families that will have to adapt to the needs of the protocol so it is important to have their views and perspectives. Separate work with the children could yield helpful information about tolerance to procedures in the study, etc.*

The group worked together for the whole day – they learnt together and avoided the 'experts know best' approach.

www.peopleinresearch.org.

Global networks

There are established patient research networks internationally in cancer, mental health and many other areas, that collect patient experiences and views, and influence what and how research is done.

The Cochrane Collaboration Consumer Network provides consumer (patient, carer, parent, etc.) input into developing Cochrane systematic reviews of best evidence in health care and in utilizing this evidence. They achieve this by being part of research review groups and contributing to conferences.

EXAMPLE: PPI IN PEER REVIEW OF RESEARCH
The Cochrane Wounds Group is based in York, UK, and
chaired by Professor Nicky Cullum at the Department of Health
Sciences. The group works with 17 health care users around
the world who act as peer reviewers and help with prioritizing reviews
for completion and updating.

INVOLVE (2009)

**EXAMPLE: PPI IN PRIORITY SETTING FOR EUROPEAN
RESEARCH**
ERA-NET PRIOMED CHILD is a European collaborative of
researchers, clinicians, parents and young people working
together to create European priorities for research aimed at improving
medicines for children. The project uses focus groups of young people
with long-term conditions to explore gaps in the research and consensus
development methods to agree priorities.

www.priomedchild.eu

EXAMPLE: PATIENT INFORMATION IN THE US

Emmi Solutions, creator of web-based interactive media,
collaborates with the American Cancer Society, a national
voluntary organization. The two parties have developed programs to
simplify complex medical information in a way that makes it easy for
patients and carers to understand.

www.emmisolutions.com/

EXAMPLE: EUROPEAN PPI RESOURCE
The European Patients Forum Value+ Toolkit is a resource for
patients and patient organizations. It provides information
on good practice relating to patient involvement in EC
projects.

www.eu-patient.eu/Initatives-Policy/Projects/ValuePlus/Resources/
Value-Resources/

Monitoring of health services

Monitoring means observing and capturing data about health care (or health care research) in accessible records that enable people to assess how well care or research is being delivered, see Figure 2.1.

Patients and the public can be the source of data to assess quality, access and relevance of services provided, but by involving them in governance we are moving towards a more transparent culture of learning for improvement and compliance.

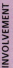
INVOLVEMENT

Public

An acute hospital trust is underperforming in two key areas: 18-week waiting list for cancer treatment and 4 hour A&E. The trust board has made these two areas performance priorities and has set up a working group. PPI is a key remit for the working group

Patients

Gather experiences of patients from A&E or cancer treatment (18 weeks). Review any existing survey work done for assessment purposes, including patient satisfaction surveys. If needed, do more discovery of patient experiences and observations

ENGAGEMENT

Public

Experienced PPI professionals work with a small group of patients providing ground rules for a transparent debate and information exchange about sensitive issues. Members of Health Scrutiny Committees attend group

Patients

Local Involvement and Cancer Support groups use information gathered by patients about quality of care in cancer services to work with the trust board

EMPOWERMENT

Public

A working group is set up by members of the trust board, local involvement and cancer groups to interview patients in A&E. Results are fed back into service delivery

Patients

Example
Providers of health care have a statutory obligation for a patient or a representative of a patient group to sit on their board as a non-executive director. In this role the patient representative will be part of the strategic decision-making process, which determines local health priorities

Figure 2.1 Monitoring of health services.

In the UK, Overview and Scrutiny Committees (OSCs) take on the role of scrutiny of the NHS, not just major changes but the ongoing operation and planning of services. They bring democratic accountability into health care decisions and make the NHS more publicly accountable and responsive to local communities.

> The NHS Alliance in the UK has started a national debate about accountability in the health services and sees PPI as one of the key ways of achieving more accountability in health and social care organisations.
>
> www.nhsalliance.org 'Whose NHS is it anyway?' A national debate on an accountable NHS (2009).

Developing health organizations

In the UK, health organizations are organized into PCTs, which need to become 'World Class Commissioners' able to shift the NHS towards a more localized, personalized, responsive and accountable system.

> **commissioning** Commissioning is the process of ensuring that health and care services provided meet the needs of the population. It is a complex process with responsibilities ranging from assessing population needs, through prioritizing health outcomes, and procuring products and services, to managing service providers.
>
> **'World Class Commissioning'** is a **statement of intent,** designed to raise ambitions for a new form of commissioning that is a **response to the significant challenge of moving power from providers to patients** or those who act on their behalf.

Commissioning requires mechanisms to help the public get involved in shaping these services and to help professionals understand the needs of populations and individuals.

Guidance on commissioning contains competencies that concern PPI, including working with community partners and, leading the local NHS. 'World Class Commissioning' suggests that care providers need to fully engage and involve patients and the public as citizens in conversations about health needs, strategic planning, service design and decision making. They must communicate with the public to increase their understanding and confidence in using local services.

There is clear evidence that health care organizations worldwide are taking PPI far more seriously than in the past. A recent national survey of PCTs in England found that leadership for PPI had climbed the organizational structure (Chisholm et al., 2007). PPI is now seen to be more a corporate job: it's everybody's business.

However, commissioning is not the sole driver for change. In Australia, the National Health and Medical Research Council and the Consumers Health Forum of Australia worked together to agree a 'Statement on Consumer and Community Participation in Health and Medical Research'. When representatives of both organizations worked together they realized that they shared issues concerning education and training for involvement and participation.

EXAMPLE: REPUBLIC OF IRELAND
In the Republic of Ireland, a Strategy for Service User Involvement in the Irish Health Service has made clear the expectation that service users will be involved in the 'planning, development, delivery and evaluation of the health services' that they provide. Year 1 of the strategy focuses on leadership of service user involvement in health service organizations.

Department of Health and Children, Health Service Executive (2008)

EXAMPLE: THE QUALITY MK PROGRAMME
(MK stands for Milton Keynes, a town in the UK with a population of around 180,000)

Quality MK is placing evidence, service users and primary care right at the heart of deciding how to deliver the best possible health services to the population (www.qualitymk.nhs.uk). It is a team made up of Milton Keynes PCT, a Patient and Public Involvement project steering group and the Centre for Evidence-Based Medicine at Oxford University (www.cebm.net).

The project has three principles:
• Engaging with clinicians in strategic planning and service design
• Public and patient engagement
• Evidence-based approach to commissioning

How PPI has affected service development within this framework:
1 A survey of public and patients (spearheaded by a patient representative), and a workshop with primary care staff led to the development and adoption of a clear pathway of action for improving alcohol misuse.
2 Care planning of diabetes enables people with diabetes to take an active involvement in deciding, agreeing and owning how their diabetes will be managed. Working in partnership with clinicians, they decide on a care plan that the patient owns and is therefore more likely to make happen.
3 Discussion between general practitioners, patients with mild to moderate depression and data from patient questionnaires contributed to a service specification that recognized the needs of patients with different degrees of depression.
4 Patient Participation Groups (PPGs) are now in all GP practices across Milton Keynes. They draw from a 'How to get started' guide produced by the Quality MK team and a PPG network (www.miltonkeynes.nhs.uk/ppg.htm)

Developing an organizational strategy for PPI

Choosing the most effective strategy for engaging the public should be based primarily on what is the intended goal of talking to patients and the public. However, other contextual factors, such as types of issue, resources or community characteristics, also shape how the public should be engaged.

A public engagement strategy should identify:
- who will be engaged
- the level of engagement
- the decision-making phase during which the public is involved.

Frameworks and criteria for evaluating public engagement strategies can help in assessing effectiveness, but no evaluation tool trumps the importance of having a clearly defined goal and strategy (Canadian Health Services Research Foundation, 2009).

Key components of a strategy should be:
- Clear goals and how PPI fits in the larger decision-making process of your organization.
- Clear links between PPI activity and organizational outcomes.
- Clear and objective supporting information for the above.
- Procedures that promote power and information sharing among and between all participants in the PPI process.
- Procedures and processes that are seen as legitimate by others.

Organizational PPI strategy table

What PPI policy affects your organization?	Who is responsible for PPI in the organization?	Who are the external challengers to our organizational PPI policy?	What PPI events does this organization deliver?
World Class Commissioning	Director of human resources	Non-executive directors	Monthly newsletters to all voluntary organizations
The Appointments Commission	Director of communications and engagement	Strategic Health Authority	Public health road shows to rural communities bi-annually
NHS Constitution	Director of medical education and training	Health Overview & Scrutiny Committee	Seminars and lectures by patient groups to staff members
Organization vision and mission statement		LINKs	

Define structures within your organization

Your own organization may have staff dedicated to involving patients and the public in some way. These may be called PPI officers or managers, patient liaison staff, patient panel or forum support staff. If your organization doesn't have a PPI function, it will probably have a Patient Advice and Liaison Service.

Known as PALS (www.pals.nhs.uk/), these have been introduced to ensure that the NHS listens to patients and carers, answers questions and resolves concerns as quickly as possible. PALS can help the NHS to improve services by listening to what matters to patients and feeding this into services management.

Define structures outside your organization

The Local Government and Public Involvement in Health Act (2007) abolished patient forums and the Commission for Patient and Public Involvement in Health, and introduced Local Involvement Networks (LINKs) in 2008. These are locality based, and should be seen as a major local resource for PPI. Run by local individuals and groups and independently supported, the role of LINKs is to find out what people want, monitor local services and use their powers to hold them to account.

Each local authority has been given funding and is under a legal duty to make contractual arrangements that enable LINk activities to take place.

LINKs organizations should aim to move communities from a position of **involvement** in health to one of **engagement** and **empowerment** to ensure that local health services are developed bottom up rather than top down.

For more information on LINKs go to www.nhs.uk/NHSEngland/links/Pages/links-make-it-happen.aspx. In 2011/12 the LINKs organization will be replaced by HealthWatch.

Four ways to develop PPI

Here are four ways of developing any PPI project:
- Climbing the ladder.
- Completing the cycle.
- Reading the map.
- Operating.

Reflect on how your organization works and which of the four fits best.

Climbing the ladder

Arnstein's ladder of participation focuses on the levels of participation, from passive to active and the shift of power to a more equitable relationship as you move up the ladder (Arnstein, 1969).

Where do your activities fit in the ladder of involvement?

Term	Activity
Is this INVOLVING? Are we informing/consulting patients or the public?	**Consultation:** to get feedback and ideas on new or existing ideas, plans, projects and services
Is this ENGAGING? Are we partnering or working directly with patients or the public?	**Research:** developing protocols, steering groups, helping with recruitment and accrual
	Services development: testing and evaluation of new ways of doing things. Will involve redesign-related groups and tasks
	Governance: being a critical friend to existing projects, providing checks and balance. Relevant for areas such as health and safety, clinical governance and complaints
	Implementation: helping in getting change through – dissemination, being part of selling a new idea, policy, service change

Term	Activity
Is this EMPOWERING? Are we placing the final decision-making authority in the hands of the patient or the public?	**Commissioning:** ensuring that local voices and experiences inform commissioning processes and plans **Research:** developing research priorities **Policy development:** working in an equitable way to develop a policy such as diversity, education and training

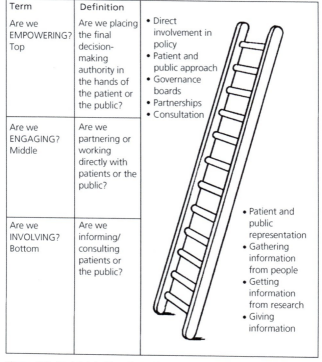

Term	Definition	
Are we EMPOWERING? Top	Are we placing the final decision-making authority in the hands of the patient or the public?	• Direct involvement in policy • Patient and public approach • Governance boards • Partnerships • Consultation
Are we ENGAGING? Middle	Are we partnering or working directly with patients or the public?	
Are we INVOLVING? Bottom	Are we informing/ consulting patients or the public?	• Patient and public representation • Gathering information from people • Getting information from research • Giving information

Figure 2.2 Arnstein's ladder of participation.

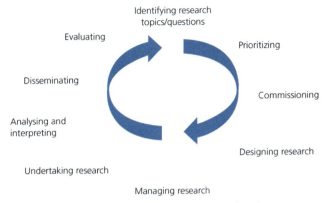

Figure 2.3 Patient and public involvement in the research cycle.

Completing the cycle
A simple **engagement cycle** could be:

- Inform patients and public about services on offer.
- Gather feedback on views or experiences of services.
- Evaluate the service using all feedback information.
- Agree any service developments with those who have a vested interest in the service.
- Inform patients and public about the changes.
- Make the changes.

The thing about a cycle is that it continues to go round – so once the changes are made a period of settling down is needed and then the review process starts once more.

Figure 2.3 illustrates the most common steps in a research programme. PPI could happen at any stage of this cycle but will more typically happen at the beginning and the end, i.e. identifying research questions and issues and early study design and then in the latter dissemination stages. There is evidence of increasing PPI in the middle part of the cycle and in some cases 'user-generated and managed research'.

Reading the map
Mapping is about understanding, visually, where you are with a process. It is used extensively for marketing and sales purposes and for organizational development.

PPI mapping could be about establishing current coverage of PPI activity in your organization or identifying areas of a service that are a priority for PPI. The map needs to describe areas of a service or function; this could be cross cutting as below or specialty specific for example children's service, etc.

Service development	Evidence of PPI	Success of PPI
Clinical outcomes		
Quality of service		
Safety and complaints		
Dignity and respect		
Information and support		
Access – place or time or both		
Continuity of care		
Discharge and aftercare		

This type of project requires some resources and a structure – it will give you a picture of how your organization is doing and help you establish where it needs to go. You could use the colour code in this toolkit to establish the depth of PPI.

Creating a map of your local groups, advocacy services and communities of interest is an important first step in PPI. Do you know what exists in your area, both geographically and in terms of your area of interest? There are plenty of potential sources of information and someone may have beaten you to it, so check with other health/social care organizations before you start.

We have used a common respiratory disease – asthma to illustrate this approach.

Status	Example	Contribution
Specific patient groups	Disease specific	Local network of parents all with children with asthma
Generic patient groups	GP practice patient group	Asthma care in primary care
Generic public groups	Toddler/playgroups Elder groups	Access to public and parental perceptions of asthma

Status	Example	Contribution
Communities of interest	Community development groups, 'green' groups, sustainable networks	Access to public perceptions of asthma
Statutory groups	LINKS NICE – Citizens Council	Focus on how asthma clinics are provided in a local community Consensus building on issues related to asthma
Voluntary/ Charitable Sector	Asthma UK Allergy UK	Prevalence incidence data to support self-care
Online Groups/ Communities	Occupational Asthma/ Alternative therapies for asthma	Anecdotal evidence Unfiltered evidence Consensus views on asthma issues Hot topics
Forums	Professionals sharing good practice in PPI	Developing knowledge and best practice
Knowledge groups	Internet home for PPI information	Networking facility Accessing examples Developing the evidence base
Membership groups	UK Royal Colleges UK Respiratory Research Collaborative (includes relevant patient groups)	Specific perspectives of asthma care and treatment Lobbying for asthma research
National groups	In Control	Championing self-management of funds for personal care
European groups	European Association of Asthma and Allergy Associations	27 organisations in 14 different countries
International groups	International Primary Care Respiratory Group	Has developed guidance for treatment and care

This can then complement the national and specialist picture. Before you start your project collect this information and think about the potential of each group to your project.

How to make a PPI map

Step 1 Why do you want to make a PPI map?

Think about: a visual summary can convey complex information quite quickly. You can show relationships, events and entities quite effectively,

Step 2 Make a list of all the organizations you know who need to be involved,

Think about: giving each organization a colour code depending on its status, e.g. voluntary organizations are green, statutory organizations are red,

Step 3 Which ones do you have personal contact with? Who has personal contact with the ones you don't know?

Think about: the quality of the relationship, e.g. a strong relationship is represented with a bold solid line and a thin broken line represents a new relationship,

Step 4 What is the relationship between the PPI organizations?

Think about: how and when and in what format the PPI organizations meet, such as committees, in public, workshops. Choose a symbol to denote format,

Step 5 Ask the group members if they think any other organization needs to be included on the map. If so add them to your list.

Think about: the best way to elicit information from patients or the public – telephone interview, questionnaire, workshop,

Step 6 Make a first draft of the map.

Think about: how easy is it to understand. Show it to someone not connected to the work to give first impressions,

Operating

This way of approaching PPI is much more about the doing of it and learning from experiences across the organization. It can be ad hoc compared to climbing the ladder, completing the cycle and reading the map, but is probably how PPI works in most organizations. For example, a member of staff has a PPI idea and implements it in their work area. They may pass on their learning to other colleagues and a gradual culture change occurs – or not! The problem with an operational approach is that it can happen in pockets across an organization and actually learning is not transferred readily and people make the same mistakes over and over.

However, there is a lot to be said for 'having a go' and experiencing PPI on a first-hand basis.

Using the operating analogy you might want to think about how this ad hoc approach can be converted into a more systematic framework using the ladder, cycle and mapping models. Choose the model which best fits the organization and project.

SUMMARY: WHAT IS PPI?
Starting any PPI project requires an understanding of:
- What PPI is and what PPI is not
- Why PPI is important in health and health research
- Why PPI is growing in importance
- PPI legislation
- How PPI impacts on health and health research organizations
- Where you, your project or your organization is on the PPI ladder

References

Arnstein S. A ladder of citizen participation. *J Am Inst Planners* 1969; **35**: 216–24.

Chalmers I. What do I want from health research and health researchers when I am a patient? *Br Med J* 1995; **310**: 1315–18.

Chisholm A, Redding D, Cross P, Coulter A. *Patient and Public Involvement in Commissioning: a survey of primary care trusts.* Oxford: Picker Institute Europe, 2007.

Department of Health and Children, Health Service Executive. National Strategy for Service User Involvement in the Irish Health Service 2008–2013. Department of Health and Children, Health Service Executive, 2008. www.hse.ie/eng/services/Publications/ Your_Service,_Your_Say_Consumer_Affairs/Strategy/Service_User_Involvement.pdf

INVOLVE. *Senior Investigators and Public Involvement.* Eastleigh: INVOLVE, 2009. www.invo.org.uk/pdfs/SIFINALPAPERNOV2009101109.pdf

NHS Constitution 2010. www.dh.gov.uk/en/Publicationsandstatistics/Publications/ PublicationsPolicyAndGuidance/DH_113613

Further reading

Ashworth R, Skelcher C. *Meta-evaluation of the Local Governement Modernisation Agenda: progress report on accountability in local government.* London: Office of the Deputy Prime Minister, 2005 (available at www.communities.gov.uk/publications/ localgovernment/metaevaluation2).

Colin-Thome D. *Mid Staffordshire NHS Foundation Trust. A review of lessons learnt for commissioners and performance managers following the Healthcare Commission investigation.* London: Department of Health, 2009.

Jenkinson C, Burton J, Cartwright J, Magee H, Hall J, Alcock C, Burge S. Patients' attitudes to clinical trials beliefs about the value of patient involvement. *Health Expectations* 2005; **8**: 244–52.

Lister, G, Jakubowski, E. Public engagement in health policy: international lessons. *J Manage Marketing Healthcare* 2008; **1**: 154–65.

Lukensmeyer C, Torres L. *Public Deliberation: a managers' guide to citizen engagement.* IBM Centre for The Business of Government, 2006.

Martin GP. Representativeness, legitimacy and power in public involvement in health-care management. Medical contributions to three illustrative conditions, and recent UK NHS policy initiatives. *Sociol Health Ill* 2008; **30**: 35–54. www.eprints.nottingham.ac.uk/ view/divisions/LSS7.html

National Institute for Health Research Central Commissioning Facility. Resources for volunteer peer reviewers. www.nihr-ccf.org.uk/site/consumerinvolvement/resources/default.cfm

The Organised Efforts of Society. ACEVO. http://www.menshealthforum.org.uk/21697-third-sector-sets-big-society-agenda

Secretary of State for Health. *Learning from Bristol: the report of the public inquiry into children's heart surgery at Bristol Royal Infirmary 1984–95.* London: The Stationery Office, 2001.

Telford R, Faulkner A. Learning about service user involvement in mental health research. *J Ment Health* 2004; **13**: 549–59.

European web link

www.euro.who.int/observatory

CHAPTER 3
How to conduct effective PPI

Patient and public involvement isn't always easy. It is helpful to think about effective PPI as being a process that is 'front loaded'. In other words, the time and energy spent at the beginning will pay dividends in the longer term.

This means thinking about:
- What you want to achieve with the involvement activity.
- How this links to health care or organizational aims, who you want to involve.
- What you envisage happening.

STARTING TO THINK ABOUT PPI

PPI is more likely to succeed where:
- PPI is considered right at the start of a project.
- There is good project management and leadership.
- The right people get involved.
- People associated with projects act as PPI champions.
- People associated with projects are able to challenge the process and decisions if they feel it is going 'off course'.
- There is a minimum of two patients or members of the public involved, taking the pressure off any one individual and maximizing the skills available to the project.
- Adequate resources are identified and provided.
- You have patience and perseverance, especially when things don't appear to be going too well.
- You start small and build up credibility in clinical, management, patient and public communities.
- There is transparency about issues in the project, e.g. politics, reducing project resources, resourcing influencing decisions, etc.
- People involved in the process feeling valued and part of a team effort.

Patient and Public Involvement Toolkit, 1st edition. By © J. Cartwright, S. Crowe, R. Perera, C. Heneghan & D. Badenoch. Published 2011 by Blackwell Publishing Ltd.

BEFORE YOU START INTEGRATING PPI ...
... you need to ask **'12 hard-hitting questions'**
 1 What are we aiming to achieve?
 2 Where have we got to so far?
 3 What will the patients and the public get out of it?
 4 Are we prepared to resource it properly?
 5 Why have we not done this before?
 6 Are we prepared to involve patients and the public from the start?
 7 Are we being honest, are we managing their expectations?
 8 What are our expectations?
 9 Are we prepared to give up some power?
 10 Are we prepared to take some criticism?
 11 What is the level of commitment to this from the top and the bottom of the organization?
 12 Are we prepared to make changes long term or is this a one-off activity/event?

Searching for literature about involvement

You must start your PPI work by finding out what has already been done in your area. This means both topic area and local area.

You should distinguish between two types of search:

1 Searching for (process) information about the process of public involvement.
2 Searching for (outcomes) information about involvement activities in your topic of interest.

Be clear in your mind, which is important to you.

Formulate a clear question for your search and use this as the basis for identifying search terms. The following will be helpful

ASPECT	EXAMPLE
PPI processes or methods that are relevant to me	Focus groups, interviews
PPI topic areas or outcomes I am interested in	Mental health; service improvement metrics
PPI setting that is most important to me	Urban acute services and crisis intervention

Searching the grey literature for PPI publications

Grey literature means reports and publications that are not produced by the usual scholarly publishing channels. It includes some very important types of document for PPI. Often, the results of involvement activities are reported in technical reports published by governments or third sector agencies, or in conference proceedings or the like.

This means that if you are serious about searching for PPI information, you need to go further than PubMed. Find out from your local librarian what databases are best for the grey literature in your topic area and in the type of organizational setting that is most relevant.

PPI search terms

There is no validated set of search terms for PPI as there is, for example, for treatment studies. However, the following search string is used by NHS Evidence: Patient and Public Involvement.

- (patient OR public OR carer OR consumer OR user) ADJ (involvement OR participation OR engagement). Other searches have been conducted using terms such as (citizens juries) or PPI or (patient & public involvement forums).
- This can be combined with your question terms to focus on PPI studies.
- Note that some databases do not use the adjacency operator 'ADJ', so you need to check the specific instructions of how to search each database.

In searching the internet using search engines, it pays to be specific. Use quotation marks to delineate phrases and include terms to describe methods, topics, outcomes and settings as noted above. Be prepared to test out different combinations though, as the internet is not as well indexed as commercial bibliographic databases.

Searching and citing issues in PPI

There are three types of articles on Public Involvement in Research.

1 Articles ABOUT public involvement in research.
2 Articles reporting research project FINDINGS.
3 Articles reporting public involvement as a METHODOLOGY.

Searching and citing issues in PPI

ABOUT	FINDINGS	METHODOLOGY
Challenges: No specific journal Editors, peer reviewers lack context and guidance Focus more on impact on individuals rather than on the research itself	Challenges: No standardized method of reporting public involvement No built-in method of tracking involvement activities throughout the research process	Confusion about meaning of terms: Public involvement Participatory research Action learning

Issues when searching for published articles
- Once research is published it is difficult to find.
- PubMed prefer terms 'consumer' and 'participation'.
- Social Care Online prefer terms 'user and 'participatory' as well as involvement.

What next?
- Encourage journals to publish both the findings of research *and* how the public were involved in the research.
- Need for researchers to be aware of the different types of impact and how to report on all of them.
- Need for researchers to be clear about who involvement benefits.
- Consider the incentives for researchers in involving the public.

Involving the right people
Once you have established what you want to achieve and how involvement will add value to this work, think about the type of people and their qualities that you need.

Qualities and attributes of involved patients and public
This is one of the most important parts of PPI: thinking about the experiences, qualities and attributes of involved patients and public that are desirable for the project. Getting this 'fit' right can make all the difference to the success of the work. Of course many people will bring more than one attribute, often people who 'wear different hats' are more able to think laterally about PPI and see possibilities and opportunities rather than barriers and problems.

Skills set – developing and nurturing individual talent
If you know the level of involvement, engagement or empowerment you are expecting from patients and the public, it will help you to identify the skills and potential of individuals.

This in turn will help you to identify their training needs. Training can be an excellent way to introduce people 'gently' to the PPI process. We return to the issue of training in Chapter 4.

DESIRABLE SKILLS
- Able to self-manage (important if they have chronic condition)
- Organized – ability to keep to timetables/commitments
- Basic literacy
- Ability to reflect
- Open minded
- Like working in a group/team
- Ability to work within a structure
- Desire to learn
- Ability to challenge
- Personable

PPI Skills and Attributes put into Practice

Level	Skills & Attributes	Contribute to	Outcome
INVOLVE	Sharing experiences, interests and views on health topics	Surveys Pathway diaries Focus Groups	Better quality and authentic patient centred date
ENGAGE	Organised Ability to challenge Ability to work with different professional groups	Developing health information leaflets Research applications Business case documents	Transparent processes Better use of health resources
EMPOWER	Presenting Decision making Chairing	Commissioning Panels Analyzing Research Data Chairing Public Forum Delivering training	Improved democratization of health services

EXAMPLE: THE JOURNEY FROM INVOLVEMENT THROUGH ENGAGEMENT TO EMPOWERMENT

Step 1: Involve

John has a child with diabetes. It was an unexpected shock when his son developed this condition. In order to seek more information about the condition John joined a national diabetes charity. Once fully equipped with information to help his son manage his condition and after a period of consolidation, he becomes frustrated at the limited delivery mechanisms for insulin. He starts to talk to colleagues about his frustrations and realizes he has an interest in research in this area and potentially has something to contribute.

Step 2: Engage

John contacts a diabetes research network and offers some of his time. Following induction he joins a study advisory group. The group is concerned with developing research ideas and assessing grant applications. He enjoys this work and sees that there are gaps in innovative research into alternative insulin delivery. Through his networks he meets a specialist research industry-based group.

Step 3: Empower

John is enthusiastic in contributing his ideas and experiences to this research group who are exploring novel ways of administering insulin. A research idea is formed and John is involved in negotiating for his original diabetes charity to become a co-bidder on the grant application. John helps to convene a focus group of parents of children with type I diabetes, to explore their experiences of insulin delivery and contribute to the refinement of the research proposal.

John becomes a named co-applicant on the research proposal and co-presents at a national conference.

Contrasting qualities and attributes of patients and public

Patient	Public
Direct experience of clinical condition	General experience of patients' conditions
Direct carer experience of a clinical condition	General experience of carers' perspective
Parents of children with a particular clinical condition	Parents of children who have used services
Recent experience of using services	General experience of service use
Experience of being involved in research, either as a research subject or as part of planning and implementing research	No experience of research
Making a complaint or feeding back on a poor service	Media representation of services
Knowledge of health services	Knowledge of local community services
Good at making links with other patients with the same condition	Good at making links across projects and bringing in others to take part

PPI methods and tools

PPI methods should be matched to the purpose of the involvement activity, your available resources and the likelihood of recruiting patients or members of the public to get involved. There are different routes to use your methods and tools: face-to-face, online/audio and paper based.

The main PPI methods are:

- reviewing documents
- surveys, questionnaires and interviews
- focus and discussion groups
- workshops and training
- exhibitions and road shows.

A voluntary organization with a focus on stroke is working with the local health service to improve local services for stroke patients via the following methods.

1 A **survey** of stroke patients, carers and stroke specialist staff will establish what they think is needed with the new service. There might also be published evidence about the configuration of effective stroke services.
2 A **workshop** will set the scene, consider the findings of the survey and set them in context of the resources available to develop the service.
3 Developing consensus about what is most important in the service (in relation to the resource allocation).
4 Feeding back to those who contributed to the survey and the event with regard to commissioning developments and outcomes.

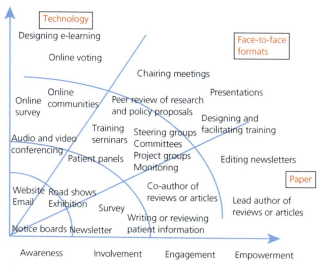

Figure 3.1 Examples of PPI using different media.

Different methods for different outcomes

There is a distinct difference between involvement activity that is consultative in nature, and PPI that has a more action-based focus. Consulting is about eliciting a wide range of public views, but with the final decision about how those views are used not being made by the public. PPI is about listening to the public and patients and working with the information they provide to influence an outcome.

Depending on the objective and desired outcomes of any PPI project, different methods need to be selected at the outset.

KEY MESSAGE
Method matches the purpose, and your resources

Levels of PPI processes

INVOLVEMENT

Consultative processes
The objective of a consultative process is to fill an information gap. You will have questions such as 'What do patients and carers think about current stroke services? What do they think can be done to improve them?'
There may or may not be pre-existing information and data to address your questions. You should ensure you review these resources prior to a consultation so that your audience knows that you are serious.
Consultation is a one-way process in which patients and members of the public supply data to fill your information gaps. Analysing this data will yield new and illuminating information about a service or health condition.

ENGAGEMENT

Deliberative processes
The aim of a deliberative process is for participants to deliberate on information, experience and views together to achieve a common goal.
Such processes are increasingly relied on to capture the range of diverse perspectives of patients and members of the public.
Deliberative processes encourage informed public debates and lead to policy recommendations that incorporate diverse points of view.
Deliberative processes that focus on concrete recommendations are more likely to have a direct influence on health care decision making.

EMPOWERMENT

Consensus development processes
A consensus development process seeks the agreement of most participants but also the resolution of mitigation of minority objections. Consensus is usually defined as meaning both general agreement and the process of getting to such agreement.
It may be used in decisions about priorities, disinvestment and rationing.
Often this will combine aspects of the first two processes. A range of patients or the public equipped with information and data need to agree areas of priority in an equitable and transparent way.
It is vital that the process is open to scrutiny because as with any form of priority setting there will be casualties, i.e. issues that don't make the priority list, so it is important for the organization to be able to account for these decisions.

Outcome	Methods	
Communicating the need for PPI activity	Local media, newsletters, online forums, posters and leaflets, exhibitions, road shows	✅
Communicating health messages		
Gathering views and experiences	Surveys, open and consultative meetings, interviews, home visits and focus groups	
Consultation on existing ideas or plans	Structured workshop with an element of consensus development or voting on the ideas or plans	
Assessing the potential impact of new services	Rapid appraisal (assessing communities and groups at risk, gathering information quickly and from the ground)	
Generating new ideas	Creative thinking workshops, focus groups, a 'suggestion box', incentives and interviews	
Synthesizing views to filter into decisions	Deliberative events and meetings, asking individual patients about their care and treatment	
Governance and probity	Membership of monitoring groups, patient or public as chair of group	
Input to information	Members of the target audience of the information must be involved at early stage of its development	
Closing the feedback loop on PPI activity	Sharing reports and plain language summaries of complex projects, feedback sessions, launch events, conferences, local media stories and profiles	
Making moral decisions about services, research	Ethics committees, research interest groups, citizen's juries, panel discussions	
Developing areas of consensus or priorities	Nominal group technique, consensus conferences, Delphi surveys	

Reviewing documents

Patients and the public can give invaluable perspectives on health care documents, such as policies, research proposals, project reports, etc. This may be as part of a panel of experts or a working group, but could also suit people who prefer to work alone or who like to be home based.

Common agreement is on the need for:

- finding out about the involved patient's/member of the public's interest and relevant skills
- describing the peer review process and paperwork – examples are helpful here
- assessing the need for specialist training (e.g. overview of research methods) and capacity to handle the task
- introducing the involved patient or member of the public to the review panel chair and observing a review panel meeting in progress (without participating)
- offering before and after follow-up on the telephone or by email to check on progress within the review committee.

EXAMPLE: PEER REVIEW
The UK National Institute for Health Research Central Commissioning Facility has useful resources that help volunteer peer reviewers to establish what is and is not helpful feedback, as well as dummy applications to work with and guidance on how to complete review forms.

www.nihr-ccf.org.uk/site/consumerinvolvement/resources/default.cfm

---

Designing a questionnaire for a survey

The aim of a questionnaire is to get as many answers as possible from the patient or public group you want to work with. This checklist will help you to maximize impact and response.

- Ensure the questionnaire has a short and meaningful title
- Keep questions short and succinct
- Use colour and design to make it visually attractive
- Offer incentives for completion
- Make it easy to return – include a stamped addressed envelope
- Ensure instructions for completion are clear and unambiguous
- Decide if you want to use open or closed questions
- Put the most important questions at the start of questionnaire
- Decide the pros and cons of sending electronically or by post
- Pilot the questionnaire before distribution to the whole sample

---

For more details about questionnaire design in a PPI context see Jenkinson *et al.* (2002).

Running a focus or discussion group

A focus group is a form of qualitative research in which a group of people are asked about their attitude towards a product, service, concept, advertisement, idea or packaging. Questions are asked in an interactive group setting where participants are free to talk with other group members.

FOCUS GROUP CHECKLIST

Action	Checklist
Step 1: Prepare focus group topic guide	• Have a clear understanding of the background to why you want to run a focus group • Read ALL the relevant literature • Prepare list of themes for discussion • Prepare individual questions under each theme • Ensure questions are short, clear and concise – for a 2-hour focus group assume rule of thumb three sides A4 questions • Test the questions out on colleagues • Avoid ambiguity
Step 2: Prepare focus group protocol	• The protocol guides how the focus group will be run • It ensures continuity across large numbers of focus groups and different facilitators • It also acts as a personal checklist and reminder, e.g. have I remembered the name badges and expenses money?
Step 3: Recruit focus group participants	• Who do you want to recruit and why? • How will you recruit them? • How many do you need to recruit? • What is the timeframe for recruitment? **Recruitment methods:** • Advertising • Community groups • Hospital lists
Step 4: Confirm focus group participants	Confirm to selected participants the following information: • date of meeting • time of meeting • venue • map

Step 5: Set up the focus group interview	• Ensure tables and chairs are arranged in a circle • Tape recorder and microphone placed centrally on table. Ensure all equipment works • Have coffee and biscuits ready on arrival • Greet participants and provide name badges • Ask participants to complete consent/demographics form • Introduce yourself, introduce participants • Explain purpose of focus group • Explain how long the focus group will last • Explain that you are keen to hear ALL views • Confirm confidentiality and anonymity of recording • Ask for permission to switch on tape to start recording discussion
Step 6: Run the focus group	**Managing participants 1:** • Ensure that each participant is allowed to express their opinions and ideas • If necessary state this to the group. **Example:** *'It is important during our discussions today that each person feels free to tell his or her own story about their experiences of hospital care'* **Managing participants 2:** • Use first names when asking a question to make individuals feel included **Example:** *'Tom, would you like to tell the group about how you benefited from rehabilitation after your triple bypass operation?'* **Managing participants 3:** • Ensure that very vocal members do not take over the discussion **Example:** *'Thank you for sharing that with us Mary, perhaps we can ask other members of the group about their experiences of emergency care. What about you Sid?'* **Managing participants 4:** • Ensure that as many themes as possible are covered **Example:** *'I think we can now move away from talking about critical care and discuss how efficiently you were discharged from hospital. Bill, can you tell us what information you were given about home care when you left hospital?'*

Use of language
- Keep questions clear and concise
- Avoid jargon
- Demonstrate empathy

Example
'That must have been very traumatic for you Jenny'
Demonstrate genuine interest. It is important that participants feel you value their views.

Step 7:
Close the focus group

- When all themes have been covered ask participants if there is anything else they would like to add to the discussions
- Thank them for attending the focus group and confirm how valuable their contribution has been

Administration:
- Hand out payment
- Complete any claim forms
- Ensure all participants leave venue. Help to transport if necessary
- Label tape. Dispatch to transcriber

Running a workshop

Tools that you could use:
- scenarios
- information packs
- visual materials
- terms of reference
- working together tool – 'tree type' icebreaker.

How to use scenarios as a PPI tool

When working with patients and the public use practical examples they can relate to in order to create meaningful engagement. A practical way to do this is by using scenarios. Scenarios give a snapshot of a situation a patient or member of the public might find themselves in.

In this example a scenario was used to help patients think about what skills they would expect a clinical nurse to have as an expert in patient education. The feedback from the patients helped to develop competences skills for clinical nurses.

USING SCENARIOS TO HELP PATIENTS CREATE CONVERSATIONS ABOUT THE QUALITY OF A SERVICE

You are a patient who has recently been diagnosed with a long-term medical condition. Together with your partner you are meeting the nurse for the first time to discuss treatment options, local support services and long-term care.

As part of the Patient Educator Project, the clinical nurse specialist will be expected to have the following **competences**:

- Enable individuals to make informed health choices and decisions
- Organize information and materials for access by patients and carers
- Work with individuals to evaluate their current health status and needs
- Agree a plan to enable individuals to manage their condition

Think about each of the competences and how they might be demonstrated in the above scenario. Try to break each competence down into:

Performance criteria – How well it must be done

Knowledge and understanding – What knowledge is needed to match the competence?

Clinical knowledge – What clinical knowledge is needed to match the competence?

Your feedback will help us to understand the skills clinical nurse specialists need to educate patients in self-care if they have a long-term medical condition.

Information for participants ahead of PPI activity

The essentials:

- The venue name, address, site map and indicate if the meeting room will be marked.
- Public transport information.
- Parking information (including the sort of change needed for pay meters).
- Information about the nature of the meeting, group, task (see briefing below).
- Claim form for travel and other payment arrangements.
- The name and contact number of someone who can help with any last-minute problems (this can be very reassuring especially at the start of a project).

Good briefing includes both general briefing, on topics such as how decision making is done, commissioning and working with evidence, as well as a specific briefing on project issues.

Where there are important papers to send prior to meetings, consider giving information that will help involved patients and the public make sense of them. These could include a front sheet that tells readers:

* what the paper is about in two sentences
* when it was written
* the author(s)
* what decision or discussion process the paper is designed to trigger
* whether there is an element of consensus needed to move forward.

In practical terms documents needed to be sent in good time, such as 7–14 days before. Send either by email or post (establish this early on; many patients won't have access to printers or be able to manage large amounts of paper). If you have an unavoidably large document consider writing a one-page summary. Consider using glossaries of commonly used terms in health care.

People briefing

People briefing is likely to rest with a good chairperson who should ensure that introductions are made, badges and names plates used, and biographies shared before meetings if appropriate.

EXAMPLE: PEOPLE BRIEFING – A MEDICAL CHARITY

On leaving HM Forces (Army) after 24 years service in 1982, we moved to London, where I worked for 20 years at the Bank of England. In 1984 or thereabouts I was diagnosed with _____, which was fairly mild, so mild in fact, that I thought I could do without medicine. Although I was put on various drugs, my _____ reminded me that I still should take the medicine.

About 8 years ago while on holiday in Germany I had a near fatal attack and it was only the quick action of my wife and sister-in-law that I believed saved my life.

Since then I joined _____ and became a 'Speaker on _____ visiting schools, Rotary Clubs, colleges, etc., giving talks. I have also been involved in many focus groups and as a patient on research panels.

While my _____ has not got any worse, and I take _____ morning and night, I do have a skin problem, _____, mainly patches on the legs and scalp, and it affects my nails.

On being made redundant in 2000, I set up a small printing and IT business from home, which I have been running ever since. I am married and have a son of 39 years, and two grandchildren.

Alternatively, you could ask participants to supply the answers to the following questions ahead of the meeting.

My name:
I am participating (cross out those that don't apply)
    As me
    To represent other people – please say who
    To represent an organization – please say which one
I have a job title and it is:
The job/role that I do is:
I can make decisions about:
I cannot make decisions about:
Special skills or knowledge that I bring are:
Things you need to know to work with me are:

Terms of reference

Terms of reference show how the scope of the work will be defined, developed and verified. They should also provide a documented basis for making future decisions and for confirming or developing a common understanding of the scope among the people involved in the group. It is helpful to have a clear picture of success factors, risks and restraints. They are important for groups of people who will meet regularly, because they promote effective team working.

Ideally the group members should develop terms of reference themselves (with some guidance about project milestones and achievements).

It is the chair's responsibility to ensure that the group works within the terms of reference. They should be reviewed regularly to ensure that they remain relevant.

PROJECT STEERING GROUP TERMS OF REFERENCE

Purpose of steering group	To ensure that the project assists health care research and service organizations to better reflect the experiences and values of service users
Context to project	There is much that is still not understood about the causes and treatment of [disease] and many different views about the best way forward. The [disease] project should increase patients' and carers' influence on the research agenda; it will provide better access to participants for researchers undertaking qualitative studies; for service providers it will create a better insight into the experiences and priorities of service users

Outputs of project	• Patient experience database • Website and virtual network • Working together
Role of the steering group	The steering group will work to: 1. **Advise** on the direction and implementation of the project 2. **Monitor** progress and ensure adherence to plan 3. Keep the project **scope under control** 4. Monitor the **project budget** and make recommendations about expenditure 5. Receive **progress** reports from the project coordinator 6. Ensure effective **communication** between partners 7. Provide a platform for considering the variety of views and **reconcile** differences in opinion 8. Encourage **cooperation** between partners 9. **Address** any issue with major implications for the project
Role of steering group members	• Be genuinely interested in the project • Work with other members respectfully and constructively • Have a broad understanding of project management issues and be able to challenge decisions • Be committed to and actively involved in pursuing the project's outcomes • Attend all meetings and be prepared to contribute

---

KEY MESSAGE
Select methods carefully. Choosing the best method to match the situation will ensure best outcomes

Practical considerations
Payment for PPI
Payment helps to incentivize people to get involved; it appeals to a wider range of potential people to get involved, especially those in more marginalized circumstances; and it acknowledges the value of involvement and promotes equity in relationships.

Quite often people don't need or want to be paid – but this should not prohibit the offer, and in this case vouchers and other thank you gestures can be greatly appreciated. Whether someone is paid or not, thanking them and feeding back the results of their involvement is essential.

Despite being an area of ongoing debate there is emerging consensus about the essential considerations, which are as follows.
- Reimbursement for expenses is not payment for skills time and expertise.
- Involved patients and members of the public should not be out of pocket for any expenses incurred during the involvement activity. This may include: travel costs, carer, childcare or personal care costs, overnight accommodation, meals and snacks.
- Payment for conference fees, training and office supplies may also apply.
- Payment for time skills and expertise may vary across organizations, but it is considered best practice. There are examples in the resource section.
- Make the payment or reimbursement as easy as possible; consider having cash available on the day for smaller amounts.
- Issue receipts for payment (a simple form will do) that are signed by both parties.

Things to be aware of with payment:
- National Insurance and personal tax
- Employment Law
- benefits and allowances
- institutional rules.

The resource section contains the most up-to-date guidance. However, the most important thing is to talk to people about their circumstances and what they feel comfortable with.

If the involvement activity is clearly described, consider a summary of this with the agreed fee for payment, reimbursement rules (mileage for example) and how the payment will be made.

Sometimes large health or research institutions don't make it easy for payment to non-employees. This shouldn't deter you from offering payment but may require some negotiation on your part to meet the institutional rules that apply.

Finally if you are planning involvement activity in a project or work stream build in costs to cover payment and reimbursement.

Venues for meetings and events

Where patients and the public meet is often overlooked in the whole process of PPI, but it has an impact on the success of any PPI event. Participants want to feel welcomed and need to leave any PPI event feeling positive.

Here are some key points to help you achieve both.
- Always visit a venue before you book it.
- Ask the venue manager to go over your specific requirements.
- Ensure the accommodation is fit for purpose, especially from a disability access point of view.
- Acoustics – do you need a hearing loop; is the venue private for sensitive discussions?

- Equipment – do you need internet access, computer and projector?
- Confirm the booking and get a contact name and number for last-minute problems.

Seating

How and where people sit is another feature of involvement work that you can positively influence. Specify the layout of the room to suit your involvement activity.

Activity	Implications
Lots of people to listen to speakers	Lecture-style seating and think about microphones
Do you want people to talk to each other?	Cabaret-style seating will enable this but cut down on your overall numbers
Do you need a smaller group to have good eye contact during discussions?	Think about a large table (preferably hollow centre as this reduces the sense of lots of wood between participants)
Something that ticks all of these boxes?	A horseshoe is a good compromise – it isn't quite lecture style and does allow eye contact for large groups of people

Creating a welcoming atmosphere

Any event is not just about gathering a group of individuals together under one roof to focus on a certain topic. It is also about creating an atmosphere and environment where individuals can do productive work together. We have all experienced social gatherings which either went like a bomb or bombed out! Thinking, planning, organizing and attention to detail are the ingredients that make a good event and should include:

- remembering the basics – shaking hands, smiling, etc.
- developing the art of enquiry when greeting participants
- ensuring that preparation is obvious, such as correct name badges
- introducing participants to each other to encourage networking. 'Take a 'who knows who' and, 'who might be introduced to who'? approach to seating.

An icebreaker: tree types

When patients, health professionals and the public come together in groups, PPI professionals need to spend time breaking down barriers to ensure that everyone works together as effectively as possible.

Sometimes the best way of achieving this is for individuals to think outside the roles they play in their everyday lives. For example, it can be helpful for a doctor or nurse to discuss issues from the point of view of being a patient rather than a professional. The use of metaphors to describe personal and work attributes can help people connect with each other without focusing on professional roles, labels and stereotypes. For example, ask people to think of themselves as trees, animals or flowers.

We have used a 'tree type' tool as an icebreaker. It is a fun, creative and engaging method of helping disparate groups work together effectively by stepping outside of their everyday roles.

What to do
1 Ask all participants to describe the characteristics of different trees.
2 Allocate each member a tree type.
3 If the group is large enough, allocate each tree type into tree groups, e.g. forest/arboretum/orchard.
4 At the start of the workshop or meeting provide each member with details of their tree type and tree group and ask them to discuss how accurately the characteristics reflect them as a person. Ask them to select a characteristic they like best and to apply that characteristic during the meeting or workshop.

EXAMPLE: 'TREE TYPE' ICEBREAKER

Tree type	Characteristics	Tree group
Apple tree	Lots of charm, appeal and attraction; pleasant attitude, flirtatious smile, adventurous, sensitive, loyal in love, wants to love and be loved; faithful and tender partner, very generous, many talents, loves children, needs affectionate partner	Orchard
Fir tree	Extraordinary taste, handles stress well, loves anything beautiful; stubborn, tends to care for those close to them, hard to trust others, yet a social butterfly; likes idleness and laziness after long demanding hours at work, rather modest, talented, unselfish, many friends, very reliable	Forest
Elm tree	Pleasant shape, tasteful clothes, modest demands; tends not to forgive mistakes, cheerful, likes to lead but not to obey; honest and faithful partner, likes making decisions for others, noble-minded, generous, good sense of humour, practical	Arboretum

www.mysticfamiliar.com/library/astrology/tree_astrology.htm

Exhibitions and road shows

PPI Exhibitions are where you have a clear message and objectives that you wish to share with a community or targeted population. The exhibition may be in a health care setting, such as a hospital or doctor's surgery, or it may be in a community centre or a college for example. A road show is where you repeat this process in different locations, perhaps to reach different audiences or to achieve some geographical spread, the emphasis here being on taking your message out to the people. A road show could comprise an exhibition, some drama or an interactive exercise such as a survey.

Road shows have particular application in rural settings, to access specific populations or where there are poor transport links to get a message out into a community. It's all about making contact with the man in the street.

Your messages have to be clear and concise to maximise the impact of your brief contact with the audience. You will need to collect contact details from the public so that people can get more involved. This is especially relevant if people cannot become part of on line communities.

CHECKLIST FOR PPI EXHIBITIONS OR ROADSHOWS

First and foremost, be clear what you want to achieve
Is it:
- conveying a message?
- getting feedback on change?
- collecting interest and local contacts?

Make sure you get noticed!
- Have striking graphics, clear messages and content and a neat, well laid out stand.
- Plenty of accessible literature is vital so that visitors to your stand can help themselves.

Layout your exhibition stand to the best effect
- Check out the amount of space you have and also, to a degree, the shape of the booth or area you have booked.
- Do not clutter your space; make your exhibit look inviting and welcoming.

Make sure your people get it right!
- Man the stand with people who are comfortable dealing with the general public or specific audiences; they need to make eye contact, establish rapport and not be intimidating.
- Make sure that your people wear name badges.
- They also need to be thoroughly briefed prior to the event, particularly in dealing with the sorts of enquiry you are likely to get.

- They should be familiar with the objectives of the exhibition and be able to answer questions about them in some detail.
- If you are collecting contacts, make sure that you capture these accurately. Most importantly, you should follow them up within a week to establish contact again, even if it is just to thank them for stopping by and giving their details and saying that you will be in touch when you have some news or developments.
- If possible, get patients and members of the public who are already involved to help out at the exhibition.

Interviews

Interviews are commonly used tools in involvement and engagement. They can provide in-depth and rich information about patients' experiences, especially for those that receive community health services. There are some basic considerations when planning interviews:

- Place and timing.
- Creating the right atmosphere.
- What is the context for the interview?
- How to capture the discussion?
- Interview questions.
- What you will do with the data?
- Follow-up after the interview.

With some conditions it is essential to think through extra considerations. A joint project in ME/Chronic Fatigue Syndrome PRIME (Partnership for Research in ME) offered an opportunity to work with people with the condition before embarking on a programme of 40 interviews. Common features include cognitive, audio and visual impairment, as well as fatigue.

Some extra pointers that came from this process included the following.

- Don't accept offers of tea/coffee from the interviewee – the effort to do this will reduce the time they are available to do the interview.
- Be prepared to interview in a darkened room.
- Be prepared to speak in a low and soft voice.
- Be prepared to conduct the interview in short snatches with breaks. This demonstrates the added value of PPI to a research process.

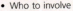 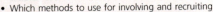

SUMMARY: HOW TO CONDUCT EFFECTIVE PPI
Developing any PPI project requires making decisions about:

- Who to involve
- Which methods to use for involving and recruiting
- Matching the best methods to suit project purpose and outcome
- How to use PPI tools effectively
- Where to deliver PPI events

References and further reading

British Medical Association. Patient Participation Groups in Primary Care (www.bma.org.uk/patients_public/ppgintro.jsp). This resource has been developed to address the role of patient participation groups (PPGs) in primary care. It can be used to prompt reflection and discussion about the role of the community in the governance of a general practice, as well as doctor–patient relationships.

Flick U. *An Introduction to Qualitative Research*, 3rd edn. London: Sage, 2006.

Jenkinson C, Coulter A, Bruster S. The Picker Patient Experience Questionnaire: development and validation using data from in-patient surveys from five countries. *Int J Qual Healthcare* 2002; **14**: 353–8.

National Institute for Health Research. Payment and reimbursement rates for public involvement. INVOLVE October 2009 (available on www.invo.org.uk/All_Publications.asp).

National Institute for Health Research. Guide to reimbursing and paying members of the public actively involved in research. INVOLVE revised August 2006, Appendix 2 updated April 2009 (available on www.invo.org.uk/All_Publications.asp).

Rapid Community Consultation and Action Planning Toolkit. Oxford: Oxford Rural Community Council, 2006 (www.oxonrcc.org.uk/media/Toolkit%20Completdf%20 for%20web1.pdf).

Scott J. Payment for involvement in research: helpful benefit rules and systems for avoiding benefit problems. INVOLVE 2008 (available on www.invo.org.uk/All_Publications.asp).

CHAPTER 4
Building relationships

Recruitment and networking

Finding the right sort of people to involve can be challenging and can often be one of the main barriers to effective PPI. You have thought about the sort of people and their attributes that will add value to your project – now you need to recruit them.

There is a cumulative effect to recruitment and networking – the more you put into it the more you will get out. If you run effective PPI projects and look after people, the word will get out locally that you can be trusted and you will then find that people and communities will help you to find more or different people to involve. Try not to think about each encounter as a one-off but more a set of ongoing relationships.

Methods for recruitment
Advertising

- Advertising in local media and free press, local authority publications, local radio.
- Advertising in local libraries, social service reception areas, GP offices, schools, colleges, post offices, etc.
- Advertising in national patient groups, umbrella organizations, existing networks.

Networking

- Disease or condition based.
- Support and self-help.
- Local involvement networks or groups.
- Welfare rights and advisory agencies.
- Advocacy.
- Faith-based groups.
- Older people/youth clubs.

Golden rules of networking

- Be prepared to go to patients and the public.
- Respect the work that they do.
- Thank them for their time.
- Make the request and your offer clear.

Patient and Public Involvement Toolkit, 1st edition. By © J. Cartwright, S. Crowe, R. Perera, C. Heneghan & D. Badenoch. Published 2011 by Blackwell Publishing Ltd.

Techniques

- Visit the group in a setting on their terms.
- Be watchful and attentive.
- Actively listen to the conversations and debate.
- Be prepared to present your idea/request.
- Think about what's in it for you and what's in it for them.
- Learn about the group before you make your pitch.

As with all recruitment activity it is worth thinking about what's in it for the involved patients and public.

The sorts of **benefit** that involved patients and the public have cited are:

- Improving services – either direct changes to a service or research to find out how to improve it.
- Improving care and treatment.
- Making research more relevant to their experiences of living with a condition.
- To challenge stigmatization.
- To advocate for under-represented groups.
- A gateway for personal development.
- A civic cause or pride.
- Wanting to 'make a difference' and/or prevent a poor experience.
- To have a meaningful role in a community.
- To earn money.

CHECKLIST FOR PATIENT RECRUITMENT AND INVOLVEMENT

- Agree type of patient group you want to recruit or involve, e.g. young people with diabetes.
- Develop a description of what you want them to do.
- Draw up a list of organizations that work with or are networked to your patient group, e.g. Diabetes UK, local PCT, GP practice.
- Contact relevant organizations and establish how they can help you recruit and involve patients, e.g. attending diabetes clinics/drop-in centres, attending workshops/forums (DAFNE), writing to newsletters.
- Meet with patient group and agree a way of working together, e.g. ground rules.
- Draw up a project plan setting out project milestones (recruitment process: purpose, person specification, time required, context/group interaction, responsibilities and accountability, level of commitment required, paperwork required, support identified, outcomes and impact of involvement, evaluation).

Support and training for participants and professionals
Participants

The most important aspect of support and training for involved patients and public is that you consider it in the first place. A good place to start is to discuss and check their understanding of the task and context of the project and if they have any concerns.

You could ask them how do they feel about it using a scale of 1–10, with1 being uncomfortable and unconfident, and 10 feeling very comfortable and confident. This will give you a helpful marker of now and also something to compare with later in the process.

You could then progress with what will make them feel better and more confident about the involvement activity. Simple activities that help include:

SIMPLE ACTIVITIES FOR PATIENTS
- Reading about it.
- Watching someone else do it.
- More information about the issue – and an opportunity to talk this through with someone.
- Spending time with others involved (especially on non-related business, i.e. getting to know each other) – especially good for a group process/activity.
- Learning or brushing up on a new skill such as appraising documents, presenting, chairing a meeting, computer skills, analysis and figure work, putting a case for change.
- Looking for information and evidence.
- Debriefing after events.
- Informal pre-meetings before the actual meeting.
- Telephone contact the day before an activity as a 'check in'.

Professionals

Of course PPI can hold some negative associations for some health care professionals. The sorts of anxiety can be around:
- fear of failure
- professional exposure
- dealing with patients who are angry or 'have an agenda'.

There are also potential issues about the integrity of the involvement activity; for example, what if the involvement activity tells us things that we don't want to hear?

Training may need to address areas concerning:
- honesty and candour
- developing trust and taking risks with each other
- knowing when not to be there and when to support patients
- understanding self (bias, influence and hang-ups).

Training resources

There are a number of resources that can help, which are set out in Figure 4.1.

For patients/public	For professionals
Information, resources and events for promoting public involvement in NHS, public health and social care research www.invo.org.uk	Provides training for public consultation www.consultationinstitute.org/home/
Patient UK www.patient.co.uk	Information, resources and events for promoting public involvement in NHS public health and social care research www.invo.org.uk
People in Research www.peopleinresearch.org	Making sense of research evidence: CASP: www.caspuk.org.uk
Folk.us Provides training events about involving people in research. www.folkus.org.uk	Hertfordshire University Module www.herts.ac.uk/home-page.cfm
Provides training and tools on the benefits of public engagement www.involve.org.uk/	Provides training and tools on the benefits of public engagement www.involve.org.uk

Figure 4.1 PPI training resources

Interpersonal skills: running effective meetings and workshops

Effective meetings need the following ingredients:
- A good chairperson or facilitator.
- Clear aim and objectives – 'by the end of this meeting we will have…'. (It is worth repeating this several times).
- Participants who understand the part they will play in this process.
- Constructive challenging of decisions and good management of conflict.
- Ensure that the rules of dignity, respect and equality of voice are adhered to – people remember how they were treated more than what was discussed.

Role of chairperson or facilitator

The chairperson or facilitator is the personal face of PPI. Their role is to get the best out of the assembled people. They are not there to share their wisdom and experiences; in fact, sometimes it is advantageous to have a chair or facilitator who is not intimately involved in the work, but is skilled at the art of enquiry.

What are good enquiry practices?

- Clear and concise questions.

- Delivered in a calm and open manner.
- Using clean language, without tone or bias.

Good inquiry demands 'observational listening'
- Content, what is being said.
- Context, how it is being said.
- Projection, why it is being said.
- Together you get more than the picture, you get the background.

Ask questions even when you know the answer
Because:
- You will find out more about the situation, e.g. context.
- You will establish what the other person knows.
- You may know the answer but not the cause.

Don't go for quick-fix solutions
Because:
- By doing so, you are trying to 'win'; therefore there must be a loser.
- You may miss the complete picture; let it unravel.
- Your suggestion may be good but not liked, an argument follows.
- Your suggestion may be wrong and you lose credibility.

To get you started
This table will help you think about good and bad enquiry practices.

Good art of enquiry skills	Example	Poor art of enquiry skills	Example
Clear and concise questions	How long have you been living with diabetes?	Ambiguous questions	This illness you were talking about where you have to inject yourself each day with insulin. You said it's called diabetes, so what's it like to have to do that then?
Delivered in a calm and open manner	Even voice tone Open body language Positive non-verbal communication Do not rush but keep focused		
Using clean language without tone or bias			Umms or ahhs or not sure! I can't believe that's what you think! No sarcasm

Dealing with difficult situations and managing conflict

COMMON EXAMPLES OF POOR BEHAVIOUR
- Has side conversations during the meeting.
- Rubbishes other people's views without suggesting anything better.
- Tries to side-track discussion with inappropriate personal experience.
- Confuses everyone with 'expert' views – jargon, statistics, their vast experience.
- Dominates discussions.
- Frequently interrupts.
- Goes on and on about the same idea.
- Is constantly negative.
- Makes seriously prejudiced comments.
- Always comes late or sends apologies.
- Does not contribute at all.
- Has 'negative body language'.
- Does not switch mobile phone or pager off and keeps coming in and out of the meeting.

There are many ways to manage these sorts of behaviour. You can choose to adopt a 'command and control' approach whereby you set the context and ground rules and ensure that they are followed. Alternatively you can use peer pressure within the group to rein in unacceptable behaviour.

As a chairperson or facilitator you can also 'lock them out' from communication by your non-verbal communication. Mute eye contact, turn away from them and purposively ask other members of the group by name to contribute. Some people new to group working may not know the 'rules' and unspoken etiquette of meetings, so you may need to guide them beforehand.

When issues under discussion are emotive, or are going round in unproductive circles, consider the approaches listed below

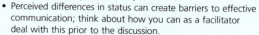

METHODS TO SOLVE AWKWARD SITUATIONS
- Separate the people from the problem.
- Perceived differences in status can create barriers to effective communication; think about how you can as a facilitator deal with this prior to the discussion.
- Use your ground rules. If the group develops these rules they are more likely to abide by them.
- Focus on interests, not positions – not 'take it or leave it' mode.

- Generate options.
- Use objective criteria so that outcomes are clear – custom and practice, law, guidelines and protocols, terms of reference, ground rules, etc.
- Never confront difficult behaviour in full glare of the group, first see if peer pressure plays a part then speak with the person privately if necessary.

Jane, an experienced facilitator in public engagement, was asked by a large commercial organization to run a series of workshops to find out what employees thought of an in-house health promotion scheme.

Her brief was to run four pre-arranged workshops with various staff members and to follow a topic guide drawn up by the human resources department. Each group had been selected according to their job roles within the organization, ranging from shop floor workers to senior management. Venues were arranged according to the status of staff members.

At the first workshop of shop floor workers, attendees were hostile towards Jane and it was clear that they did not want to take part in the process of engagement. Jane sensed that there was a great deal of anger in the room and felt that unless this anger was dealt with the workshop could not take place.

After physically tearing up the topic guide and agenda in front of the attendees she said that they each had 5 minutes to tell her why they felt hostile and at the end of 30 minutes if nobody wanted the workshop to continue that she would cancel it and they could all go back to work.

Having allowed participants an opportunity to talk honestly this is what she discovered:
1 Participants had been told to attend the workshop rather than being offered the choice of attending.
2 Shop floor workers felt less valued than their managerial counterparts because of the choice of venue.
3 Human resources had drawn up the topic guide without consultation with staff, so they felt the questions had a hidden rather than open agenda.

Knowing this, Jane focused the rest of the workshop on addressing the barriers to communication within the organization and the workshop had a positive outcome. Managing the conflict led to engagement.

Being inclusive

As chair person or facilitator be very aware of your need to include the whole group in discussions. You may need to encourage some more than others, or shut down people who dominate.

Always finish agenda points with an opportunity for final comments and observations and make eye contact with those who are struggling to contribute to encourage them to participate.

Consider using written suggestions and ideas for those who find talking in groups challenging. Encourage paired discussions as an alternative to whole group talking. Meetings tend to be more formal then workshops, consider the level of formality that you want or need and plan accordingly.

Placing of participants

People's physical position in a room can affect how they participate in number of ways:

- People with greater status may want a prominent position in a group.
- People who are unwilling to participate or disagree with the premise of the meeting may 'lurk' at the fringes.
- People who are shy or lack confidence may seek to 'hide' at the back.
- Other things to watch out for include practical things such as light, accessibility, audio loops, microphones, projector and power sockets. No one wants a laptop cable over their head or to have to crane to see a screen.

As facilitator, it is your job to make sure that these dynamics don't derail your aim. There are a number of steps you can take.

- In advance of your meeting, you should consider the mix of people and plan where you think it would be good for everyone to sit.
- Try and weigh up the value of letting people develop their own seating plan, or being more deliberative and managing who sits where.
- Do set out your space and seating to maximize eye contact and communication.
- Ensure that everyone in the group is participating well. For this, you'll need to have a good seat, where you can see (and be seen by) everyone.

You might experience some competition for this position in the room. 'Controlling' people usually want good eye contact with all participants. This may undermine the chair person or facilitator's role, so it is important you get there early to get the best seat in the house.

Allowing groups to develop

One of the most popular ways of allowing groups to develop is to refer to the **Forming – Storming – Norming – Performing** model of group development. This way of understanding group dynamics was first described by Bruce Tuckman in 1965. He maintained that these phases are all necessary and inevitable in order for a team to grow, face up to challenges, tackle problems, find solutions, plan work and deliver results.

Forming The initial and important stage when group members get to know one another, exchange some personal information and see how each other work as individuals and as a member of a group.

Storming This is where group members contribute to their ideas and experience, sometimes in harmony and sometimes in conflict. Energy levels are often high as are expectations for the process. This stage needs careful chairing or facilitation.

Norming The group enters a more settle stage often agreeing rules, values, shared methods, working tools and even taboos. Trust will begin to develop as group members become more acquainted with each other and the work in hand.

Performing Motivation and knowledge levels are high and this is when projects can start to deliver their expected outcomes. Group members are now competent, and the group can handle the decision-making process without too much intervention.

This is by no means a template for group development and there are many models in the theory of group working, but it does give an indication of likely group behaviour. Changes to structure and group composition can revert groups to earlier, less productive behaviour.

Allowing groups to develop is an important feature of PPI. Efforts at the start of the process and meetings, and workshops that help people get to know each other *as people*, helps the overall dynamic of group interactivity and effectiveness. The tools mentioned in this toolkit could all be used to help team development.

Reading the room
Whether running a meeting or workshop, a skilled facilitator spends most of their time 'reading the room'. This means that they are noticing what is going on between people without any words being spoken. They are looking for non-verbal cues to help them know what to do next.

The art of good listening
The first skill that you can practise to be a good listener is to:

> Act like a good listener

Our faces contain most of the receptive equipment in our bodies, so tilt it towards the person you are listening to. You can be a better listener when you *look at the other person*. By looking at the speaker, your eyes will also complete the eye contact that speakers are trying to make with you.

When you have established eye and face contact with your speaker, you must then react to the speaker by sending out non-verbal signals. Your face must move and give the range of emotions that indicate that you are following what the speaker has to say.

If you find yourself drifting away, change your body position to help refocus and concentrate.

If you are really listening intently, you should feel tired after your speaker has finished. Effective listening is an active rather than a passive activity.

Be aware of the following blocks to listening.

> • **Comparing**: 'when that happened to me'
> • **Mind reading**: trying to guess what the other person is really thinking or feeling
> • **Rehearsing:** what you will say next
> • **Judging**: you don't listen because you have already made up your mind
> • **Dreaming**: only half listening because something that they have said triggers a memory for you
> • **Advising**: you are the great problem solver, searching for the solution to their problems
> • **Derailing**: changing the subject and taking the conversation off in another direction
> • **Being right**: you cannot hear the criticism; if you cannot admit mistakes, you cannot change

Non-verbal communication

Non-verbal communication, including 'body language', means conveying information through conscious or sub-conscious gestures, movements or facial expressions. It is an essential aspect of interpersonal communication

The study of non-verbal communication is a complex field. In this section, we provide brief guidelines.

> **Hands** convey many messages and can be the most mobile parts of your body when communicating. Avoid pointing and jabbing; making fists (they represent forcefulness and power), 'chopping motions' and 'windmills' are very distracting for other people. Generally, palms facing away from you represents rejection and cupped palms or palms facing towards you represents inclusion and acceptance.
> **Body posture** is also important to get right. Avoid 'closed' gestures such as crossed arms or legs and turning away from your clients or colleagues. Putting your hands on your hips can be seen as pompous and slightly aggressive.

Connecting with people is vital to engage them and make them feel comfortable and secure. Eye contact is the main tool here; consciously look at the people you are engaging with – but don't stare them out!

Your appearance matters. It's not about impressing people, but feeling comfortable in yourself and not wearing items that seriously distract.

Mirroring the person you are communicating with. For example if they have become quiet and contemplative then you need to respect this and choose the opportune moment to ask a question or prompt more discussion. The trick is to differentiate between what is thinking and what is boredom. If you think that they are bored or have lost interest, albeit momentarily, then ask a question, take a break/breather, set them a short task.

Be aware of the non-verbal signs if you spot signs of dissent/ disagreement/confusions/boredom then act on it appropriately. Don't delay; they will be relying on you to read the signs.

Source: *Body Language* David Lambert and The Diagram Group, 2004 Collins.

Remember! If words and non-verbal messages conflict we take the non-verbal message as more significant.

EXAMPLE: PPI IN RANDOMIZED CONTROLLED TRIALS

Tina was chairing an advisory group set up to monitor a randomized controlled trial. Most of the members of the advisory group had either a medical or academic background and were very familiar with attending meetings. Two members of the group were patients with no medical or academic experience, but lots of experience of either being a patient or caring for a patient.

Tina noticed that from the outset that the patient members of the group were quiet and not contributing and that the more experienced members were taking the lead in the discussions.

Tina started to ask the patient members their views, in a language and tone that was inclusive, to draw them into the discussion. She also asked the clinicians to explain all medical terms in an easy to understand fashion.

By doing this Tina was setting the ground rules for engagement to be all-inclusive rather than expert-led.

Avoiding the pitfalls

In any PPI project, how you communicate with your collaborators outside of meetings is just as important as how you talk to them face to face.

In this section we will look at some of the common pitfalls and provide you with tools and suggestions for ensuring effective communication.

Common communication barriers

Communication barriers can arise at every stage of the communication process and have the potential to create misunderstanding and confusion. Never forget that for many (though not all) members of the public, getting involved in health services or research means getting to grips with some alien terminology and unfamiliar methods.

Some common barriers include:

- Your message is too lengthy.
- Your message is disorganized or contains errors.
- Poor verbal communication and body language.
- Providing too much information too fast.
- Your message takes no account of your participants' culture or context.

To be an effective communicator and to get your point across without misunderstanding and confusion, your goal should be to lessen the frequency of these barriers at every stage of the process.

Use the following with clear, concise, accurate, well-planned communication as follows.

- Who are the participants?
- What are their needs?
- What is their health literacy?
- How can I use visual aids to enhance understanding?

This is especially important in PPI work where you may be communicating with a diverse range of participants with diverse needs.

TOP TIPS FOR EFFECTIVE COMMUNICATION

- Tell it like it is
No one really likes spin; integrity and willingness to tell the truth are very valuable commodities.
- If you really believe it, show it
More and more people believe only what they can see happening with their own eyes in their own world. So say and then do.
- Listen before you think or speak
Active listening is where you make a point of finding out what people think rather than making assumptions. Strangely, people who've listened first, tend to get listened to when they speak.
- Headlines first, then the whole story

Attention spans are short, get your main message in first; attention will be sustained if it is something that benefits them.
• Consistency is the clearest message
If you do the same thing again and again people will notice, understand and trust you to do the same thing in the future.
• If it really matters, do it face to face
Email is like broadcasting in that you never really know when or whether people are taking notice.
• Involvement is the best persuader
If you want real understanding then you need to get people involved, in the debate, the discussions, decisions or delivery.
• Encourage feedback and act on it
If you pay lip service to feedback you'll quickly stop getting it. The more that you act on feedback and are seen to act on feedback (note that both are necessary), the more feedback people will give you.
• Little and often is better than long and loud

Online communication in PPI

The past 20 years have seen a revolution in communication via telecommunications, computing and media.

THE BENEFITS OF ONLINE COMMUNICATIONS TO PPI
• Currency of information
• Ease of access, input and retrieval
• User-generated content
• Instant communication
• Mobile technology

One key benefit of online communication is the possibility for interactive, user-generated content to feed into the health and care agenda. Users can interact with organizations, and with each other, in different ways. This has particular benefits for PPI, as it opens new channels through which to understand people's views and experiences.

There are key accessibility benefits too. These come in the form of online diaries and narratives, blogs, newsletters and e-communities.

In planning online involvement, you need to consider the following.
• Do you have the technical and design capacity to set up and maintain the system? If not, consider outsourcing these functions.

- Things to ask about outsourcing solutions include: do they provide adequate support? Do they have experience in the health and PPI context?
- Have you committed time and effort to managing the input you receive? Online communities don't just happen spontaneously. You need to put effort into promoting awareness, training and support for users, responding quickly to queries and making sure discussions stay focused.
- Can you make sure that people do not misuse the process (e.g. for malicious complaints)? You must be prepared to deal with difficult feedback and establish a transparent process.
- Do you have a way of validating the data you receive (i.e. making sure that people don't 'spam' you with just one side of the story)?
- Can you demonstrate that you are taking note of the feedback and acting on it?

Teleconferencing etiquette

This is often referred to as conference calling or audio conferencing, and refers to any conference that takes place via a telephone. The key etiquette rules that apply to phone teleconferences are as follows.

A round of introductions is necessary	The very first thing that should take place before a teleconference call begins is to introduce all of the conference call participants. Everyone should have a clear understanding of who is present in the room listening in on the call. If there are many participants, the chair should them to introduce themselves whenever they speak
Reduce all possible distractions	Conduct the call away from the distraction of noise generated by colleagues, phones and keyboards
Be considerate	This is just as important in personal meetings as it is in conference calls. Let others speak. Don't interrupt. Don't monopolize the conversation so that no one else has the opportunity to voice an opinion
Keep an eye on time	Set a time limit on the conference call when you organize the conference so that everyone can plan accordingly. Don't allow the conference call to get off topic. Stick to the agenda. If you find yourself going over the time limit, be considerate. You may need to postpone the rest of the conference call until a later time to accommodate everyone's schedule
Finishing off	When particular points have been covered, check back with participants for any final comments or observations before you move on (much harder to judge this when working telephonically)

Videoconferencing

This is a practical option for people who have limited mobility or who are housebound. It is also very cost-effective, especially with dispersed groups. Its utility can also apply to global patient groups.

Active desktop presentations

This is a group activity, which is led with a presentation. All group members log into a given website and either Skype or teleconference in additionally. It allows audio and visual connection. Participants can watch a demonstration or presentation, read documents and view programs that are run on the computer of the host. It is usually possible to 'switch' host, so that someone else can show participants what is on their screen.

You can find plenty of advice on videoconferencing and related technology etiquette online. Search for 'etiquette' and the technology you are planning to use, or start at www.emilypost.com/business/video_conference.htm

Communicating by email

Email etiquette is rather more diffuse, as different people regard emails differently, and of different levels of formality. Some useful rules of thumb for PPI email communications are:

- Think before you write – send a message that will be clear and useful.
- Be accountable for your message – you never know where it may end up.
- Remember that email is not always confidential and may end up in the public domain.
- Consider when to 'cc' others into emails.
- Indicate on emails whether documents are shared for information or for action.
- Take time to proofread it before you send it.
- Keep your message concise.
- Do not type in capitals, it looks like yelling.
- Do not type in all lower case.
- Bear in mind that people may vary in their response times to emails.
- Just because you sent it, doesn't mean they've read it: check for error messages and ask for an acknowledgement of receipt if it is important.
- Are you using the right 'signature' at the foot of your email?

Communicating in advance

To make the most of any meeting, teleconferencing or workshop some preparation time will pay dividends on the day because:

- It makes clear why the meeting/workshop is taking place and ensures clarity of purpose.
- It gives people time to think in advance about what and how they can contribute on the day.
- It allows any detailed information to be digested and understood rather than having just a brief overview or in fact the wrong view of why the meeting/workshop is taking place.
- It acts as an early 'meet and greet' message from the event organizer and will encourage attendance.

CASE STUDY: THE TRIME PROJECT (WWW.TRIME.ORG.UK)

The following exercise demonstrates how to communicate a task in advance of a workshop. The TriMe project ran a PPI research workshop where mental health patients and carers were asked about their concerns about being involved in a mental health clinical trial. The feedback was used to inform the development of a clinical trials website for patients.

Introduction to the TriMe Workshop

Getting involved in a mental health clinical trial is like going on a journey. At different stages of the journey participants will want and need information to help them along the way. We would like to know what questions you might ask on the journey to help us design the TriMe website.

What We Would Like You to Do

Look at the following table with these headings:

- **Before the trial starts**
- **When the trial starts**
- **During the trial**
- **When the trial ends**
- **After the trial ends**

Under each heading in the table, we would like you to write the most important question you would like answered at that point of the participant's journey. Here is an example to help you.

Before the trial starts	When the trial starts	During the trial	When the trial ends	After the trial ends
Q: What is a clinical trial?	Q: Why do I have to give informed consent to take part in the trial?	Q: What about if I decide to drop out of the trial after it has started?	Q: What will the researchers now do with the data they have collected from the trial?	Q: When will the new treatment be available to patients after the trial ends?

KEY MESSAGE
The public and patients are people. Treating all people with courtesy and respect as you yourself would wish to be treated, underpins the ethos of good PPI

The collaborative work brings the public a better and easier understanding and awareness of clinical trials. My involvement prompted a local NHS trust review of Clinical Trials Guidelines.
U Hla Htay, carer

SUMMARY: BUILDING RELATIONSHIPS
Developing and building relationships is a key component of a successful PPI project. When developing any PPI project it is important to know:
- How to recruit and network
- How to support training for participants and professionals
- How to run effective meetings and workshops
- Different communication methods

Further reading

Argyle M. *The Psychology of Interpersonal Behaviour*. London: Penguin, 1994.

Collette P. *The Book of Tells*. London: Bantam Books, 2004.

Coulter A, Entwistle V, Gilbert D. *Informing Patients*. London: Kings Fund, 1999.

Duman M. *Producing Patient Information: how to research, develop and produce effective patient information*. London: Kings Fund, 2003

Goleman D. *Working with Emotional Intelligence*. London: Bloomsbury, 1999.

Oppenheim AN. *Questionnaire Design*. London: Continuum, 1992.

Osborne H. *Health Literacy from A–Z: practical ways to communicate your health message*. Sudbury, MA: Jones & Bartlett, 2004.

Rodenburg P. *Presence*. London: Michael Joseph, 2007.

Withers B, Lewis, KD. *The Conflict and Communication Activity Book*. New York: AMACOM, 2003.

Useful web resources

Health Literacy Resources & Case Studies: http://smartpatientweb.org/Health_Literacy_Resource.html

Information Standards: www.theinformationstandard.org/

On-Line Engagement: www.speakup.dialogue

The Care Quality Commission involvement website: www.cqc.org.uk/getinvolved.cfm

The Patient Information Forum: www.pifonline.org.uk

The Patients Association: www.patients-association.com

Public engagement http://www.investinengagement.info/98

CHAPTER 5
Evaluation of PPI

There are plenty of people in health care who think that PPI is a 'good thing' and there are also those that feel it is a waste of time. Who is right?

Only evaluation and monitoring will tell us if PPI has made an impact on a service, patient information or the design of a clinical trial.

Historically in PPI the focus has been on getting the **process** right (and this toolkit reinforces that) because it is important, but it takes the focus away from the **impact** of involvement. For example, if we did not have PPI would we have a different result? What is the added value of PPI?

A review of existing evaluation frameworks by the Canadian Health Research Foundation (2009) shows that evaluation tools, while helpful, should not be relied on as a sole method of assessing the effectiveness of any public engagement strategy. Clearly defining the underlying goals of public engagement, and measuring results against those goals, is crucial to evaluating its effectiveness. There is also a case for building the knowledge of PPI within your organization.

Research
There is evidence to suggest that PPI increases recruitment to all types of research, in particular clinical trials, where it has also helped it improve trial design and the use of relevant outcome measures. PPI benefits the people involved in the research process, both participants and the research team.

Creating an evidence base for PPI
There is a limited amount of evidence about the impact of PPI. This is in part due to the diverse activity of PPI, the lack of structure and guidance on reporting PPI in peer-reviewed journals, and the tendency to report results rather than lessons learnt.

Strengthening the evidence base for PPI
There needs to be more consistent and robust methods for assessing the impact of PPI and finding useful means of telling the story of involvement. This story needs to be told not only by patients and the public, but also by research and health service professionals and leaders.

Why evaluate PPI?
PPI is still a relatively new area of practice within health and social care and research. It is a fast-growing area and new ideas and approaches from

Patient and Public Involvement Toolkit, 1st edition. By © J. Cartwright, S. Crowe, R. Perera, C. Heneghan & D. Badenoch. Published 2011 by Blackwell Publishing Ltd.

communities and local groups are being adopted by PPI leaders. However, PPI has to add value to a process if it is to be accepted as a credible and useful contribution to service development and research – even if there is a moral imperative at play. For an organization to invest time, resources and energy in PPI it should be interested in and critical of the outcomes of this activity. This chapter suggests ways that organisations can evaluate PPI.

Evaluating PPI methods and process

Evaluating PPI can be achieved through informal and formal research into how people work together and what they achieve. Materials and processes for working together can be examined; the interactive and participatory process can be observed by participants or by independent observers; and interviews, focus groups and surveys can gather experiences and opinions. The findings can be shared with the organization and/or participants along the way in order to improve how they work together; or they can be shared afterwards when judging the success of a completed exercise.

Examples of evaluating a PPI process

The type of questions you might be interested to include:
- How much did partners feel that their contributions had been heard and acknowledged?
- Was recruitment fit for purpose; was the group or the individual the right choice?
- Did people feel welcomed and valued as a group, team member or partner?
- How clear was their role in the exercise or process?
- How did they rate the support for their involvement, both formally such as induction, training/briefing and informally?
- What was the quality and timeliness of supporting information?
- How was the follow up from meetings and activities?

Capturing and recording involvement activity is an important part of process evaluation. If you have *not* recorded basic details such as how many people attended the workshop for example, it makes reporting on the process very difficult. In addition it is helpful for individual participants (professionals and patients/public) to record their involvement activity and reflect and feed back on how effective it was.

EXAMPLE: THE INVOLVEMENT PORTFOLIO
Developed by NHS Research and Development Forum Service User and Carer Working Group. The portfolio holder can record their involvement and participation experiences, training events, taking part in committees, etc. It encourages portfolio users to reflect on levels of involvement and skills learnt.

www.rdform.nhs.uk/docs/involvement.doc

Evaluating the impact of PPI on a service or project

There is a growing body of research evaluating the impact of PPI in health care and health care research. However, there is still little consensus on what is measurable in PPI, so much so that a recent Delphi study that asked: 'Can the impact of public involvement on health and social research be evaluated?' provided a complex picture.

The participants considered that it was feasible to evaluate the impact of public involvement on the impact issues below. *The percentage of the Panel (N=?) that rated each impact issue between 7 and 9 is highlighted in bold:*

1 Identifying topics to be researched **(83%)**
2 Prioritizing topics to be researched **(86%)**
3 Disseminating research **(88%)**
4 The member(s) of the research team **(81%)**
5 The member(s) of the public involved in the research **(92%)**

There was much less consensus around design and management in research and collecting and analysing data.

Source: Boote *et al.* (2006).

The United Kingdom Clinical Research Collaboration (UKCRC) evaluated the impact of PPI on strategic decision-making groups (boards) and concluded that PPI helped by:

- asking what may appear to be simple or obvious questions, but which are actually questions fundamental to the debate
- keeping a discussion grounded
- monitoring performance and recognizing good performance
- promoting issues or questions that members believe would be important to patients and the public
- acting as a reminder of patient and public accountability
- bringing in knowledge from other related experiences
- contributing to practical decisions
- promoting the use of plain English
- lobbying for more PPI within particular activities.

This report also acknowledged and identified some barriers to the impact of PPI:

- The complexity and context within which patients and the public were operating.
- The speed at which decisions have to be made.
- Whether PPI is core to the business of an organization.
- Lack of clarity about the role of involved patients and public.

• The politics of working together (in this case the UKCRC Board).
Source: TwoCan Associates (2009).

Evaluating the impact of PPI on the people who took part

This could be an important part of your evaluation. What have the involved patients and public found out about themselves in the process, how has it changed them, are they ready for a new challenge and can they move into other areas of PPI to assist your organization, or others?

There are several studies that suggest that there are benefits for patients and the public in involvement. These include self-worth, confidence, developing practical and new skill sets, enthusiasm for research, service development, moving into work, the satisfaction of making a contribution and helping to improve services.

Among many of the benefits was my hands-on experience of a ground breaking evaluation. I learnt much about research and the wide variety of ways in which people from very different backgrounds could work together successfully... Working in a mixed team of academics, researchers and people from a service user background was really stimulating and it was great to see in practice how much mutual respect and sharing knowledge enriched the whole project.
Angela Barnard, service user researcher

Impact on researchers and service managers

Positive benefits include the following.
• A better knowledge and understanding of the community.
• Enjoyment and satisfaction.
• Career benefits.
• Challenges to belief and attitudes.
Negative impacts include the following.
• Higher demands on resources and slower pace of research.
• Loss of power.
• Forced changes in working practice (although new skills could be see as a benefit).
• Challenging researchers values and assumptions.
Source: Staley (2009).

What is the potential impact of PPI within organizations?

PPI is the way we work here
In the local health economy PPI used to be an extra and often they didn't get round to it. Now we work together and PPI is seen as important, so we just do it.
John Needham, Milton Keynes LINk

If PPI is not 'built in' to organizational culture, there is a danger that PPI can become marginalized or fail. PPI should appear in organizational structures, vision statements and business plans. From there they need to be lived on the ground.

The Healthcare Commission has a very clear view of what constitutes useful organizational PPI.

- Strengthen the culture of being open and responsive to local people, through strong management and clinical leadership that ask people how their health services can serve them better, and act on their responses.
- Increase the influence that underserved groups of patients, users of services and the public have on the decisions they make. Trusts should also find ways of showing how engaging with people is supporting improvements to services and to people's experiences of care.
(*Listening, Learning, Working Together*, 2009)

How PPI can impact within an organization

- Creates a robust link between the mainstream health system and people who want or need to use the health services.
- Increases knowledge and understanding of a health or social condition.
- Increases knowledge and understanding of communities and people that live with health or social conditions.
- Develops alliances and networks.
- Democratizes health.

What to do to make impact happen

1 Maintain Relationships

Many people think that PPI is a one-off event. It is not. Successful PPI is about developing and maintaining relationships and networks over a long period of time. This takes time, effort and focus. Make a PPI **map** to help you illustrate the state of the PPI relationship at the start and end of a project and agree a **cycle** of engagement to ensure relationships are maintained (see Chapter 4).

KEY MESSAGE
Make a key person responsible for PPI within the organization

---

Having a focal point and person for PPI is important in larger organizations. Involved patients and the public highly value a central point of contact and a human face to PPI.

2 Practise evidence-based PPI

At the very least, evidence-based PPI process must:

- be explicit

- acknowledge bias in the process and try to minimize it
- be transparent
- be based on the best quality methods
- report clearly and openly so that others can critically appraise its methods and impact.

3   Events and profile

Regularly organize and deliver PPI events on behalf of your organization. This can be a road show about a new health service or health promotion activity. Keep the profile of PPI going with regular newsletters and blogs.

4   Follow-up

Taking responsibility for PPI at different levels within an organization will ensure maximum follow-up after the project has ended. This could involve reporting the outcomes of research and the quality of a new health service after implementation.

5   Transparency

Making sure that all PPI activities are transparent is imperative if PPI is to become embedded in organizational culture. To achieve this ensure that PPI meetings/workshops have public access and that all information is easy to access via public websites.

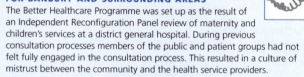

EXAMPLE: THE BETTER HEALTHCARE PROGRAMME FOR BANBURY AND SURROUNDING AREAS

The Better Healthcare Programme was set up as the result of an Independent Reconfiguration Panel review of maternity and children's services at a district general hospital. During previous consultation processes members of the public and patient groups had not felt fully engaged in the consultation process. This resulted in a culture of mistrust between the community and the health service providers.

The Better Healthcare Programme was created with an ethos of 'working together', and has delivered all of its meetings in public using webcast facilities to reach a wide audience. It also created a website to provide public access to all programme documents, reports and minutes to ensure greatest transparency.

www.oxfordshirepct.nhs.uk/news/better-healthcare/default.aspx

Once a degree of transparency has been achieved, agencies seem more willing to share capacity and control and partners who had previously been marginalised in the decision making process were more likely to play a central role.
Dobbs and Moore (2002)

CHAPTER 5: EVALUATING PPI
Evaluating any PPI project requires:
- Understanding the methods and processes available to successfully evaluate
- Understanding the impact of PPI on the service/project
- Understanding the impact on patients and the public
- Translating evaluation outputs into organizational culture

References

Boote J, Barber R, Cooper C. Principles and indicators of successful consumer involvement in NHS research: results of a Delphi study and subgroup analysis. *Health Policy* 2006; **75**: 280–97.

Canadian Health Services Research Foundation. Public engagement (Part III): how is it done? How can we tell if it's effective? *Insight into Action* 2009; Issue 53 (www.chsrf.ca/other_documents/insight_action/html/ia53_e.php).

Dobbs L, Moore C. Engaging communities in area-based regeneration: the role of participatory evaluation. *Policy Studies* 2002; **23**: 157–71.

Listening, Learning, Working Together. A national study of how well healthcare organizations engage local people in planning and improving their services. London: Commission for Healthcare Audit and Inspection, 2009.

Staley K. *Exploring Impact: public involvement in NHS, public health and social care research*. Eastleigh: INVOLVE, 2009 (www.invo.org.uk/Publications_Search.asp).

TwoCan Associates. *An evaluation of the process and impact of patient and public involvement in the advisory groups of the UK Clinical Research Collaboration. Final Report*. UKCRC: London, 2009.

Further reading

Black N, Jenkinson C. Measuring patients experiences and outcomes. *Brit Med J* 2009; **339**: b2495.

Boynton PM, Greenhalgh T. Selecting, designing, and developing your questionnaire. *Brit Med J* 2004; **328**: 1312–15 (www.bmj.com/cgi/content/extract/328/7451/1312).

Department of Health. *High Quality Care For All: NHS next stage review final report*. London: Department of Health, 2008.

Department of Health. *You're Welcome Quality Criteria: making health services young people friendly*. London: Department of Health, 2007 (www.dh.gov.uk/en/Publicationsandstatistics/Publications/PublicationsPolicyAndGuidance/DH_073586).

www.viewpointlearning.com

CHAPTER 6
The future of PPI

As patients and the public seek greater accountability from the providers of health services, the PPI agenda should aspire to become embedded in organizational and professional culture. As this happens involvement will shift to engagement and empowerment, allowing patients and the public to be fully engaged with the providers of health and social care.

This cultural shift comes at a time when global economies are considering their public finances, so the need to keep patients and the public informed about changes and cuts to services is an imperative. However, when considering what to prioritize, PPI-supported initiatives will come under scrutiny as to whether they represent value for money, can demonstrate measurable impact and have an evidence base.

This chapter will consider the impact of involvement moving to engagement and how the shift can help health services and the health research agenda. It also considers how PPI policy might evolve and develop over the next decade.

Maintaining public and patient commitment to the NHS while managing tighter budgets and rising demand will be a delicate balancing act. The NHS has huge public support, but this could evaporate rapidly if financial pressures are seen to be directly cutting services or damaging patient care. The public may also have little tolerance of commissioners or providers who have not seized opportunities to reduce expenditure and waste... Public confidence will be undermined if commissioners and providers do not present a united front, or if there are differences between PCTs working in the same health economy.
Harvey et al. 2009

How can PPI help health services and health research?

More conversations are taking place to encourage patients and public to design and deliver services together with professionals. The idea that the users of health services are a hidden resource, which can be used to transform services, is gaining ground. Here are some of the ways PPI might help in future decision-making and policy development.

Patient and Public Involvement Toolkit, 1st edition. By © J. Cartwright, S. Crowe, R. Perera, C. Heneghan & D. Badenoch. Published 2011 by Blackwell Publishing Ltd.

Allocation of resources and better use of resources

With resources in the public sector either static or diminishing, PPI can help develop consensus, provide transparency of decision making and establish the rationale for where to put limited resources. For example, an analysis of the Expert Patient programme showed that it reduced visits to GPs consultations by 7% and to A&E by 16%, saving between £27 and £58 per avoided consultation, before prescription costs, and £84 for each patient diverted from A&E (PSSRU, 2007; Leatherman and Sutherland, 2007).

If patients self-allocate their resources, through direct payments and personal health budgets, they are empowered with more choice, and receive personalized and improved quality of care. This process aims to ensure that there is a better fit with individual health and care needs. In the UK this aspect of health policy will grow, and there is a similar growth in advocacy and representative groups available to help patients and service users negotiate the system. Similarly, the role of health and care managers will include a brokerage element. For example social workers will be trained to help with self-assessment and choosing appropriate services with patients and service users.

Personal health budgets are in development and piloting phase in the UK health system until 2012. The principles are the same as Self Directed Support programmes in social care and will apply to patients that have long-term conditions and complex needs for treatment and care.

EXAMPLE: IN CONTROL
The In Control model of self-directed support has the following features.
Realistic: making the best use of the current level of resources
Universal: applicable to everyone who needs support, whatever their situation or preferences
Liberal: allowing people to choose from the full range of possible services or other forms of support
Achievable: providing practical solutions to local communities and leaders
Legal: working within the most helpful interpretation of current legislation

www.in-control.org.uk/home

EXAMPLE: BETTER USE OF RESOURCES

Nurse-family partnership programmes in the US have been evaluated over 15 years. They were found to reduce child abuse and neglect by 48%, arrests of the children as teenagers by 61% and incorrigible behaviour by 90%. It translates into benefits worth five times the investment and a saving in public spending of about $41,000 per child involved.

www.nursefamilypartnership.org

PPI in Commissioning

Commissioning in the NHS is the process of ensuring that the health and care services provided effectively meet the needs of the population. It is a complex process with responsibilities ranging from assessing population needs, prioritizing health outcomes, procuring products and services, and managing service providers.

World Class Commissioning

In the UK, primary care trusts (PCTs) are required to develop World Class Commissioning (WCC) as a method of proactively seeking and building continuous and meaningful engagement with the public and patients to shape services and improve health so that decisions are made with a strong mandate from the local population and other partners'

EXAMPLE: SURVEY RESULTS FOR WORLD CLASS COMMISSIONING

Forty per cent of PCTs in England concluded that although some were enthusiasts for World Class Commissioning (WCC), most were reluctant to attribute their positive organizational PPI changes to WCC alone, often stating that the framework coincided with or reinforced a shift towards more engagement that was already under way locally.

World Class Commissioning requires that proactive, continuous and meaningful patient and public engagement should drive commissioning decisions. The 'significant' or 'sweeping' organizational changes that many PCTs say they are putting in place may bring this goal closer, but it is not yet a reality.

PCTs are more aware of the need to get the public involved early in decisions, but also report they are far from achieving that. They are only beginning to

> *use diverse methods to reach wider circles of the community. They face a key*
> *challenge in getting their own front line staff and clinicians to engage patients*
> *and feed into commissioning priorities.*
>
> Picker 2009 (www.pickereurope.org)

Practice-based commissioning

Practice-based commissioning allows groups of family doctors to develop better services for their local communities. Patient participation groups help provide a feedback mechanism in this process.

EXAMPLE: PPI IN COMMISSIONING
Neurological commissioning support: a collaboration of neurological patient groups work alongside primary care trusts and local authorities to ensure that the needs of people living with long-term neurological conditions are met through commissioning.

www.csupport.org.uk/

Accessibility of services

There are tensions between locally provided services close to communities and specialist services provided regionally or even super-regionally. When decisions are made about sites and levels of service, PPI is essential to assess acceptable levels of accessibility, usability and quality.

EXAMPLE: THE COMMUNITY PARTNERSHIP FORUM FOR THE BETTER HEALTHCARE PROGRAMME
The Community Partnership Forum worked with hospital managers, clinicians and primary care commissioners to develop accessible children's and maternity services to meet the health needs of the local population.

www.oxfordshirepct.nhs.uk/news/better-healthcare/default.aspx

Health professionals working with patients and the public

For users of health services to work together with professionals, the training of professionals must change, so that they are able to operate in a more flexible way. PPI invites the public into the professional realm of health services and health research, opening up processes and challenging cultures, particularly hierarchies and vested interests. This is often difficult for professionals to embrace, particularly if they have been educated by the 'doctor knows best' methods. PPI can help to break down the barriers between patients and the public and professionals and assist in the process of change management. The challenge is for professionals to view patients and the public as a resource for health systems rather than a drain on the health system.

In 2008 the Post Graduate Medical Education Training Board (PMETB) organized a workshop with patients and medical professionals entitled 'Training in partnership: shaping the future of postgraduate medical education and training in the UK'. The workshop contributed to the shaping of postgraduate medical education and training of future doctors in the UK.

www.pmetb.org.uk/fileadmin/user/Content_and_Outcomes/Working_group_reports/Patients_Role_in_Healthcare_working_group_report20080620_v1.pdf

EXAMPLE: ST GEORGES UNIVERSITY MEDICAL SCHOOL AND LEONARD CHESHIRE DISABILITY
Disabled people work with first and second year medical students to challenge stereotypes of disabled people to challenge future practice. This involves shadowing each other in workplaces and attending presentations.
Source: Taylor, 2008.

Developing trust and credibility between the public and health organizations

PPI helps to build trust between health service organizations and communities and health researchers and the public. However, to embed this within health organizations, for example, they need to:

- learn from reviews
- use quality improvement data appropriately
- see complaints as a service improvement tool
- recruit board members with PPI expertise
- make links with the communities they serve
- conduct board meetings in public.

EXAMPLE: LIVERPOOL BIG HEALTH DEBATE
Liverpool PCT used multiple methods including: online ballot box, visits to community groups, events, survey and a road show, to develop its 'outside-of-hospitals' strategy. They checked the effectiveness of their methods by surveying participants at the end of the process, asking them had their views been taken into account and did the strategy reflect their views.

www.liverpoolpct.nhs.uk

Improving quality of care and reducing harm

Organizations use lots of ways to improve care: collecting mortality and morbidity data, conducting good clinical research and implementing the findings, providing feedback mechanisms on services to name but a few. PPI is increasingly becoming mainstream in all of these methods; however, perceptions and experiences of what constitutes quality of care and harm still differ between health professionals and patients and the public.

EXAMPLE: PATIENTS COLLECTING DATA
Patient Opinion is an independent website that allows members of the public, patients and carers to share their own experience of health services and hospitals and gain support from others. The stories and comments posted are passed on to the relevant NHS trust which uses the data in three main ways:

- to plan how to develop and improve services
- to give doctors, nurses and managers a feel for what patients are saying about the service they manage
- as part of the evidence that every hospital has to submit each year to show the Healthcare Commission that the hospital uses patient views to improve services.

www.patientopinion.org.uk

EXAMPLE: ORGANIZATIONS COLLECTING DATA

Patient Reported Outcome Measures (PROMS)

Currently all NHS patients who are having hip or knee replacements, varicose vein surgery or groin hernia surgery are being invited to fill in PROMs questionnaires. The NHS is asking patients about their health and quality of life before they have an operation, and about their health and the effectiveness of the operation after it. This will help the NHS to pilot and develop measurement processes that will help target areas for development and improve the quality of care.

There is some debate about the value of these measures; some clinicians believe that the data are mostly concerned with league tables. Some patients are worried that the measurements aren't sensitive enough about their particular experiences.

www.nhs.uk/nhsengland/proms/Pages/PROMs.aspx

EXAMPLE: PATIENTS WORKING WITH PROFESSIONALS COLLECTING DATA

OMERACT

One research network is trying to address these issues. OMERACT stands for Outcome Measures in Rheumatology. It is an informal international network for working groups and gatherings interested in outcome measurement across a spectrum of rheumatology intervention studies. OMERACT holds consensus conferences every two years in various parts of the world, and members of the Patient Liaison Group take part in these discussions. By having people with rheumatology conditions involved, common agreed outcome measures in trials reflect patient experiences and priorities.

www.intermed.med.uottowa.ca/research/omeract/

SUMMARY: THE FUTURE OF PPI

Over the coming years the following issues will affect the PPI agenda.

- Allocation of resources and better use of resources
- Accessibility to services
- Health professionals working with patients and the public
- Developing trust and credibility between health organizations and patients and the public
- Improving quality of care and reducing harm

Final thoughts

There is a balance between investing energy and resources in PPI processes and keeping focus on the added value and outcomes that PPI brings to health services and research. In public services generally, there is a move towards co-production, which is central to the process of growing the core economy. It goes well beyond the idea of 'citizen engagement' or 'service user involvement' to foster the principle of equal partnership. It offers to transform the dynamic between the public and public service workers, putting an end to 'them' and 'us'. Instead, people will pool different types of knowledge and skills based on lived experience and professional learning (Harris and Boyles, 2009).

Conclusions

In the future, for the PPI agenda to become one of empowerment with assertive citizens taking centre stage, there needs to be a substantial evidence base to demonstrate that PPI makes a difference and how it does this. Better evaluations and measurement on the impact of PPI will persuade funders of the economic validity and business case for PPI. As health service and health research leaders embed PPI in not only their organizational but also their own professional culture, PPI will become a strategic intent at the highest level. We hope that this toolkit can encourage a new generation of PPI professionals to get excited about the work they do and re-energize those seasoned professionals who are already on the PPI journey.

References

Harris M, Boyle D. *The Challenge of Co-production*. London: NESTA and new economics foundation, 2009 (www.nesta.org.uk/library/documents/Co-production-report.pdf).

Harvey S, Liddell A, McMahon L. *Windmill 2009. NHS response to the financial storm*. London: Kings Fund, 2009.

Leatherman S, Sutherland K. *The Quest for Quality in the NHS: refining the NHS reforms*. London: Nuffield Trust, 2007.

PSSRU. *Unit Costs of Health and Social Care*. London: PSSRU, 2007.

Taylor A. St George's' slays the stereotypes. *Community Care* 2008; 22 May.

Further reading
Community engagement

Fisher B. *Whose NHS Is It Anyway?* NHS Alliance, 2009 (www.nhsalliance.org).

Mariam KH, Oakley P (eds). *Community Involvement in Health Development: a review of the concept and practice*. Geneva: World Health Organization, 1999.

www.communities.gov.uk/documents/communities/pdf/actionplan

www.idea.gov.uk/health

www.nice.org/uk/guidance/index.jsp?action=byID&o=11929

www.nice.org.uk/nicemedia/pdf/PH009CommunityEngagementQuickRefGuide

Measuring patient experience

Coulter A, Fitzpatrick R, Cornwell J. *The Point of Care: measuring patient's experience in hospital: purpose, methods and uses.* London: Kings Fund, 2009.

http://mrw.interscience.wiley.com/cochrane/clsysrev/articles/CD003974/frame.html

Commissioning

Chisholm A, Redding D, Cross P, Coulter A. *Patient and Public Involvement in Commissioning: a survey of primary care trusts.* Oxford: Picker Institute Europe, 2007.

Department of Health. *World Class Commissioning Competencies.* London: Department of Health, 2007.

PatientView. *Local Healthcare Commissioning: grassroots involvement?* A report prepared for the Royal College of Nursing and National Voices, 2009 (www.nationalvoices.org.uk/sites/default/files/RCN%20NV%20LHC%20Report_0.pdf).

Redding D. Commissioning for public engagement. *Brit J Healthcare Manage* 2009; **15**: 408.

Medical training

Postgraduate Medical Education Training Board. Patients' role in Healthcare – the future relationship between patient and doctor, 2008 (www.pmetb.org.uk/fileadmin/user/Content_and_Outcomes/Working_group_reports/Patients_Role_in_Healthcare_working_group_report20080620_v1.pdf)

Quality Improvement

Davies E, Cleary PD (2004) Hearing the patient's voice? Factors affecting the use of patient survey data in quality improvement. *Qual Safety Health Care* 2004; **14**: 428–32.

Department of Health. *Listening, Responding, Improving: a guide to better customer care.* London: Department of Health, 2009 (available at www.dh.gov.uk/en/)

Useful web resources

International Alliance of Patient Organisations: www.patientsorganisations.org/

www.expertpatient.co.uk

www.pickereurope.org/

Index

Note: 'PPI' refers to 'Patient and Public Involvement'

Patient and Public Involvement Toolkit, 1st edition. By © J. Cartwright, S. Crowe,
R. Perera, C. Heneghan & D. Badenoch. Published 2011 by Blackwell Publishing Ltd.